Springer-Verlag Berlin Heidelberg GmbH

Peter Teller
Hermann König
Ulrich Weber
Peter Hertel

MRI Atlas
of Orthopedics
and Traumatology
of the Knee

With a Foreword by Bernd Hamm

With 324 Figures in 603 Separate Illustrations
and 17 Tables

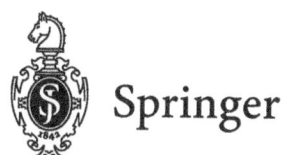

Springer

Dr. med. Peter Teller
Radiologische Praxis, Kernspintomographie
Helene-Lange-Str. 11, 14469 Potsdam, Germany

Priv.-Doz. Dr. med. habil. Hermann König
Radiologische Gemeinschaftspraxis, Kernspintomographie
Hirschlandstr. 99, 73730 Esslingen, Germany

Prof. Dr. med Ulrich Weber
Chairman, Orthopädische Universitätsklinik und Poliklinik
der Freien Universität Berlin
Zentralklinik Emil von Behring der Stiftung Oskar-Helene-Heim
Walterhöferstr. 11, 14165 Berlin, Germany

Prof. Dr. med. Peter Hertel
Chairman, Abteilung für Unfallchirurgie, Martin-Luther-Krankenhaus
Akademisches Lehrkrankenhaus der Humboldt-Universität Berlin
Caspar-Theyß-Str. 27 – 31, 14193 Berlin, Germany

Translator: Bettina Herwig, Innstr. 28, 12043 Berlin, Germany

Title of the Original German Edition:
MRT-Atlas Orthopädie und Unfallchirurgie – Kniegelenk
ISBN 978-3-540-44034-5

ISBN 978-3-540-44034-5

Cip Data applied for

Die Deutsche Bibliothek – CIP-Einheitsaufnahme
MRI atlas of orthopedics and traumatology of the knee : with 17 tables / P. Teller ... With a foreword
by B. Hamm. [Transl. by Bettina Herwig]. - Berlin ; Heidelberg ; New York ; Hong Kong ; London ;
Milan ; Paris ; Tokyo : Springer, 2003
  Dt. Ausg. u.d.T.: MRT-Atlas Orthopädie und Unfallchirurgie
  ISBN 978-3-540-44034-5   ISBN 978-3-642-55620-3 (eBook)
  DOI 10.1007/978-3-642-55620-3

http://www.springer.de

© Springer-Verlag Berlin Heidelberg 2003
Originally published by Springer-Verlag Berlin Heidelberg in 2003

Cover design: Frido Steinen-Broo, Pau, Spain
Typesetting: Fotosatz-Service Köhler GmbH, Würzburg, Germany

Printed on acid-free paper   SPIN: 10889163   21/3150/op 5 4 3 2 1 0

Foreword

With the technical advances made in MRI technology and the wider availability of MRI units, this diagnostic modality has by now undoubtedly gained a crucial role in joint imaging. The excellent detail recognition of MRI provides views of the various joint structures once only available through direct arthroscopic and surgical procedures.

The acceptance, usefulness, and role of any diagnostic modality, however, critically relies on the experience, clinical expertise, and dedication of those who use it. With this in mind, a renowned interdisciplinary team of authors have brought together expert knowledge from their respective fields in compiling this MRI atlas.

Peter Teller and Hermann König are two highly experienced MRI radiologists with backgrounds in both clinical work and research. Ulrich Weber and Peter Hertel are two leading orthopedic surgeons and traumatologists in the fields of joint surgery/microsurgery and sports injuries.

It is the vast radiologic experience in the interpretation of complex image information – an experience that takes into account the clinical requirements from the perspective of orthopedic surgeons and traumatologists – as well as the authors' didactic approach that make for the singular character of this book.

Berlin, November 2001

Bernd Hamm, MD
Professor and Chairman
Department of Radiology
Charité Medical School
Humboldt-Universität zu Berlin

Preface

MRI of diseases and injuries of the head, neck, and spinal column has become firmly established as a diagnostic tool since examiners could easily apply their previous experience gained in CT to MRI in these areas.

A similar level of experience for assessing the highly complex joint structures has not yet been reached on a large scale despite the wider availability of MR imagers and an increasing demand for such examinations.

This is due to two factors: On the one hand, the unfamiliar projections of MRI in all spatial dimensions along with the many variable imaging parameters result in a virtual flood of imaging data. On the other hand, there is a multitude of pathologies that affect the joint.

For these reasons, we came to feel the importance of presenting a format which would facilitate the formation of engrams for the major joint structures and help to differentiate clearly and effectively between normal MRI appearance and early disease.

In compiling this atlas we have focussed on the presentation of carefully selected series of MR images for each of the major joint structures ranging all the way from normal appearance and discreet changes to more severe damage and full-blown disease. The presentation of the images is supplemented by a critical discussion of the MRI findings from a clinical perspective with information on established grading systems and diagnostic pitfalls as well as their role in therapeutic decision making.

The MR images selected for this atlas (600 images representing 325 cases) have been systematically compiled over many years and have in part been presented in MRI courses. All cases have been very thoroughly revised and correlated with clinical histories, radiographs, findings at arthroscopy and surgery, and, where available, histology reports.

This reassessment revealed discrepancies in only 7.4% of the diagnoses, most of which involved the grading of severe ligamentous injury (where differentiation of extensive partial tears from complete tears of the cruciate or collateral ligaments was problematic) and postoperative imaging (in patients having undergone anterior cruciate ligament reconstruction or partial meniscectomy). Only rarely did discrepancies occur in the initial assessment of the menisci and in cases of pathology difficult to assess by arthroscopy.

With the exception of some cases displaying certain characteristic features, specific tumor diagnosis requires histologic confirmation. Contrast-enhanced imaging is rarely required in examining the joint area. Its benefit is almost exclusively limited to the assessment of inflammatory involvement and tumors and is not necessary in imaging purely degenerative disorders or traumatic injury.

The majority of images presented were acquired on a 1.0-Tesla MR imager (Siemens Impact). Units with lower magnetic field strengths also yield adequate images but the poorer signal-to-noise ratio may impair detail recognition, something which primarily affects the assessment of small structures such as the menisci.

Interdisciplinary cooperation combining the experience of radiologists, orthopedic surgeons, and traumatologists will undoubtedly make most use of the high diagnostic yield of MRI for the benefit of our patients.

While respecting the different views of our specialties we have nevertheless taken this chance to join our various backgrounds in order to achieve a unified interpretation of MR images contributing to the advancement of this technology.

Potsdam, Esslingen, Berlin, November 2001   The authors

Contents

Abbreviations

SE   Spin-echo sequence: frequently used standard sequence for MRI of all areas of the body

GE   Gradient-echo sequence: allows for rapid imaging, 2D and 3D acquisition, most suited for imaging organ areas with moving structures and for assessing articular cartilage

T1w   T1-weighted sequence, emphasizes tissue structures with short T1 relaxation times such as fat

T2w   Purely T2-weighted sequence, emphasizes tissue structures with long T2 relaxation times such as fluids

T2*w   Gradient-echo sequences with a low excitation angle produce relative T2-weighting. It is designated as relative T2-weighting because T2* is the T2 relaxation time as changed by field inhomogeneities

rho-w   Spin-density- or proton-density-weighted sequence, emphasizes tissue structures with a high proton content

FAT-SAT   Fat-suppressed sequences eliminate interfering fat signals and enhances water signal, e.g. when water and fat are mixed as in bone marrow edema

3D acquisition   Direct 3-dimensional image acquisition, allows for generation of specific views and image reconstruction

↑↑↑   High signal intensity

↑↑   Intermediate signal intensity

↑   Low signal intensity

0   No signal

1 Patellar Tendon

1.1 Technique and Method

Comfortable positioning of the knee with particular attention paid to any limitations of knee extension. Comfortable supportive padding of the adjoining parts of the thigh and lower leg and especially of the ankle joint.

Routine MR imaging comprises axial and sagittal planes. Sagittal images, at least, should be obtained with both T1- and T2-weighted sequences. Slice thicknesses of 3–4 mm are recommended. Images are to be acquired in all cases using the MR imager's circular or asymmetric extremity coils.

1.2 Anatomy

The patellar tendon constitutes the most distal extension of the quadriceps femoris mechanism. Its main fiber bundles originate from the distal pole of the patella and connect the patella, a sesamoid bone embedded in the quadriceps tendon, to the tuberosity of the tibia. Some superficial fibers of the patellar tendon pass over the front of the patella and blend into the quadriceps tendon.

In adults the patellar tendon is approximately 5–6 cm long, 2–3 cm wide, and 0.5 cm thick. A synovial sac, the deep infrapatellar bursa, is interposed between the tendon and the upper portion of the tibial tuberosity directly above the tendon-bone junction.

The height of the patella is determined in relation to the length of the patellar tendon. Under normal conditions the patellar tendon length is roughly equal to the length of the patella.

Deviations from normal patellar height (patella alta/baja) are mainly classified using the ratio proposed by Insall and Salvati (1971) (greatest patellar tendon length divided by greatest longitudinal diameter of patella). A ratio of $1 \pm 20\%$ is considered normal, while a ratio of less than 0.8 indicates a low-lying patella and a ratio greater than 1.2 a high-riding patella.

1.3 Normal MRI Appearance

The normal patellar tendon has well-defined margins and low or absent signal intensity in all sequences. It is clearly delineated against the rather hyperintense infrapatellar fat pad (unless fat suppression techniques are used).

1.4 Pathomechanism

The bony attachments of the patellar tendon may be secondarily affected by local anomalies of ossification of the tibial plateau or – less frequently – of the lower pole of the patella as in, for instance, Osgood-Schlatter disease and Sinding-Larsen-Johansson disease, respectively.

Both conditions are self-limited anomalies of ossification of unclear etiology so far having been classified as juvenile osteochondronecroses. Current knowledge, however, suggests that osteochondronecrosis in the strict sense is not present.

Other common causes of patellar tendinosis at the bony attachments are local degenerative changes and/or mechanical overuse (athletes) as the quadriceps femoris is the most powerful muscle in the human body.

Given the extraordinary tensile strength of the patellar tendon, it is assumed that rupture of this structure typically occurs on the basis of pre-existing damage (rupture mostly in the second half of life, local cortisone effects, bilateral rupture may occur).

1.5 Pathophysiology

Active Osgood-Schlatter disease manifests with tumorlike cartilaginous hyperplasia or abnormal ossification such as fragmentation in the area of the anterior, tongue-shaped portion of the proximal epiphysis of the tibia.

Active Sinding-Larsen-Johansson disease is characterized by fragmentation of the lower pole of the patella with deformation or ectopic ossification possibly persisting into adulthood.

The persistence of an accessory ossification center of the patella in the mature skeleton indicates a bipartite patella, which itself is a normal variant without disease status. The location of such an ossification center in the inferior patella corresponds to type 1 bipartite patella as classified by Saupe (1921/22).

A bipartite patella principally results from arrested development with incomplete fusion of physiologic ossification centers. Five types are distinguished, the most common involving the superolateral patella.

Chronic overuse syndromes lead to irritation of the patellar tendon, mainly of its infrapatellar portion ("jumper's knee" – patellar tendinitis), presenting with pain and tenderness of the anterior knee.

The patellar tendon typically ruptures near its proximal origin (inferior pole of patella) while medial or distal ruptures are rare.

1.6 MRI Signs of Abnormal Findings

Variants

The normal patellar tendon is roughly equal in length to the greatest patellar length. Pronounced lengthening of the tendon relative to the greatest patellar length results in patella alta (except when the tibial insertion of the tendon is abnormally deep), shortening in patella baja. Lengthening or shortening alone is typically not associated with additional intratendinous signal changes (Figs. 1.1 – 1.4).

Tendinosis of Distal Attachment in Abnormal Apophyseal Ossification of Tibial Plateau/Persisting Apophysis

Isolated bone fragment with normal bone signal anterosuperior to the tuberosity, either within posterior distal patellar tendon segments or at the posterior margin of the patellar tendon. The presence of reactive edema or bursal involvement is indicated by hypointensity on T1-weighted images and hyperintensity on relative T2-weighting (Figs. 1.5 and 1.6, Figs. 1.14 – 1.18).

Tendinosis of Distal Attachment in Schlatter's Disease

Reduced signal of tibial apophysis on T1-weighted images and increased signal on relative T2-weighting in early disease (normal radiograph), progressive disease with involvement of the patellar tendon indicated by local hyperintensities on relative T2-weighting. Advanced disease characterized by fragmented appearance of the apophysis with discontinuities and increasing signal intensity of patellar tendon near its distal insertion (Figs. 1.7 – 1.13).

Tendinosis of Proximal Attachment in Abnormal Patellar Ossification/Ossification Center of Inferior Patella

Isolated bone fragment at the lower pole of the patella with normal bone signal. May be associated with thickening of patellar tendon attachment and local intratendinous hyperintensities in both sequences (Figs. 1.36 and 1.37).

Tendinosis of Proximal Attachment in Sinding-Larsen-Johansson Disease

Signal decrease of the lower pole of the patella on T1-weighted images and increased signal on relative T2-weighting during puberty (much less common than Schlatter's disease). May be accompanied by reactive irritation of proximal patellar tendon portions with corresponding signal changes.

Inflammatory Processes/Overuse Reactions

Marked thickening of patellar tendon attachments, in particular at the lower pole of the patella (with normal bone contours and signal), producing hyperintensity in both sequences: *patellar tendinitis* or *jumper's knee*, typically seen in basketball players, jumpers, and hurdlers. Other parts of the patellar tendon may show focal signal increases as well, depending on the presence of relevant factors, and there may even be hyperintensity throughout the tendon (Figs. 1.22 – 1.26, Figs. 1.38 – 1.44).

Traumatic Changes

Mild damage with focal intratendinous areas of increased signal intensity; more severe trauma indicated by partial disruption of continuity with larger areas of hyperintensity and increasingly pronounced thickening; complete rupture possibly associated with discontinuity of the tendon and retraction as well as intrabursal hemorrhage (Fig. 1.7, Figs. 1.19 – 1.21, Figs. 1.26 – 1.35).

1.7 Clinical Role of MRI Findings

The so-called osteochondronecroses (Sinding-Larsen-Johansson, Osgood-Schlatter) only require conservative management during florid disease, even when the clinical presentation is impressive (pseudotumorous swelling at the tibial tuberosity).

Most cases can be managed by short-term immobilization with subsequent abstaining from athletic activities until shortly before skeletal maturity. Surgical measures are rarely indicated and if so, must be delayed until after maturity has been reached (caveat: surgically induced growth disorders, e.g. genu recurvatum).

Type 1 bipartite patella (isolated ossification center in inferior patella) and other forms of bipartite patella must be differentiated from patellar fractures (clinical presentation, CT, MRI).

Tendinosis of the tendon attachments of the knee (about 5% of all attachment tendinoses, about 40% of all tendinoses in competitive athletes) can be diagnosed with a high degree of certainty by positive MRI findings in combination with the requisite clinical presentation.

The decision for surgery may be difficult to make, especially in patients who are unwilling to abstain from sporting activities.

The demonstration of patellar tendon rupture is an absolute indication for surgery.

Table 1.1. Characteristic signal intensities

	T1w	T2w	T2*w	rho-w	FAT-SAT
Tendons	0	0	0 – ↑	0	0
Fatty tissue	↑↑	↑	0 – ↑	↑↑	0
Compact/spongy bone	0	0	0	0	0
Marrow (yellow)	↑↑↑	↑ – ↑↑	0 – ↑	↑↑	0
Muscle tissue	↑	↑	↑	↑↑	↑
Effusion (serous)	↑ – 0	↑↑↑	↑↑↑	↑ – ↑↑	↑↑↑
Hemarthrosis	↑↑	↑↑	↑↑	↑↑↑	↑↑

0 No signal; ↑ low SI; ↑↑ intermediate SI; ↑↑↑ high SI.

Further Reading

Bernicker JP, Haddad JI, Lintner DM, DiLiberti TC, Bocell JR (1998) Patellar tendon defect during the first year after anterior cruciate ligament reconstruction: appearance on serial magnetic resonance imaging. Arthroscopy 14 (8): 804–809

Insall J, Salvati E (1971) Patellar position in the normal knee. Radiology 101: 101–104

Johnson DP, Wakeley CJ, Watt I (1996) Magnetic resonance imaging of patellar tendonitis. J Bone Joint Surg Br 78 (3): 452–457

Kartus J, Lindahl S, Stener S, Eriksson BI, Karlsson J (1999) Magnetic resonance imaging of the patellar tendon after harvesting its central third: a comparison between traditional and subcutaneous harvesting techniques. Arthroscopy 15 (6): 587–593

Khan KM, Bonar F, Desmond PM et al. (1996) Patellar tendinosis (jumper's knee): findings at histopathologic examination, US, and MR imaging. Victorian Institute of Sport Tendon Study Group. Radiology 200 (3): 821–827

McLoughlin RF, Raber EL, Vellet AD, Wiley JP, Bray RC (1995) Patellar tendinitis: MR imaging features, with suggested pathogenesis and proposed classification. Radiology 197 (3): 843–848

Miller TT, Staron RB, Feldman F (1996) Patellar height on sagittal MR imaging of the knee. AJR Am J Roentgenol 167 (2): 339–341

Pomeranz SJ (1997) Gamuts and pearls in MRI and orthopedics. MRI-EFI Publications, pp 159–161

Popp JE, Yu JS, Kaeding CC (1997) Recalcitrant patellar tendinitis. Magnetic resonance imaging, histologic evaluation, and surgical treatment. Am J Sports Med 25 (2): 218–222

Reiff DB, Heenan SD, Heron CW (1995) MRI appearances of the asymptomatic patellar tendon on gradient echo imaging. Skeletal Radiol 24 (2): 123–126

Saupe E (1921/22) Beitrag zur Patella bipartita. Fortschr Röntgenstr 28: 37

Schweitzer ME, Mitchell DG, Ehrlich SM (1993) The patellar tendon: thickening, internal signal buckling, and other MR variants. Skeletal Radiol 22 (6): 411–416

Shalaby M, Almekinders LC (1999) Patellar tendinitis: the significance of magnetic resonance imaging findings. Am J Sports Med 27 (3): 345–349

Sheehan FT, Zajac FE, Drace JE (1999) In vivo tracking of the human patella using cine phase contrast magnetic resonance imaging. J Biomech Eng 121 (6): 650–656

Fig. 1.1. Patella baja
(41-year-old male)

Sagittal T1: Length of patellar
tendon reduced by slightly over
1.5 cm compared to greatest length
of patella, resulting in slightly lower
patellar height than normal with
prominent inferior patellar pole
(Insall-Salvati ratio 0.56)

Fig. 1.2. Patella alta
(24-year-old male)

Sagittal T1: Length of patellar
tendon increased by 1.5 cm relative
to greatest length of patella, resulting in high-riding patella
(Insall-Salvati ratio 1.31)

Fig. 1.3. Abnormal patellar tendon
insertion/deep distal insertion
into hypoplastic tuberosity
(28-year-old female)

Sagittal T1: Insertion of patellar
tendon below distal end of tuberosity. Pseudoexostosis of anterior surface of tuberosity with slight signal
decrease. Concomitant irritation of
deep infrapatellar bursa (*arrow*)

Fig. 1.4. Normal signal intensity of patellar tendon and tibial plateau apophysis, slight patella alta (11-year-old girl)

Sagittal T2*: Patellar tendon and tuberosity of low signal intensity. Minute triangular area of increased signal indicating deep infrapatellar bursa with normal fluid volume

Fig. 1.5. Patellar tendinosis of distal insertion; chronic deep infrapatellar bursitis (32-year-old male)

Sagittal T2*: Increased signal of distal patellar tendon, especially in posterior aspect, and hyperintense, increased fluid volume of deep infrapatellar bursa (*arrow*)

Fig. 1.6. Isolated ossification center of tibial apophysis – no Schlatter's disease (11-year-old girl)

Sagittal; *left* T1, *right* T2*: Small isolated bone fragment at tip of tuberosity, separated from tuberosity by a delicate cleft (*arrow*). Normal bone signal

Fig. 1.7. Abortive Schlatter's disease/local sequela of contusion (13-year-old girl)

Sagittal; *left* T1, *right* T2*: Mild signal decrease in distal aspect of tibial plateau apophysis and somewhat more pronounced decrease in adjacent anterior margin of tibia on T1-weighted image with local signal increase on relative T2-weighting (*arrows*)

Fig. 1.8. Early Schlatter's disease (13-year-old girl)

Sagittal; *left* T1, *right* T2*: Signal decrease of tip of tuberosity on T1-weighted image with local signal increase on relative T2-weighting (*arrow*). Corresponding signal changes of distal end of patellar tendon

Fig. 1.9. Schlatter's disease (11-year-old girl)

Sagittal; *left* T1, *right* T2*: Compared to preceding case, tibial tuberosity shows larger area of decreased signal intensity on T1-weighted image with signal increase on relative T2-weighting (*arrows*). Corresponding signal changes of distal patellar tendon likewise more extensive. Slightly increased fluid volume of deep infrapatellar bursa with increased signal on relatively T2-weighted image

Fig. 1.10. Schlatter's disease (13-year-old boy)

Sagittal T1: Extensive signal reduction of tibial plateau apophysis on T1-weighted image

Fig. 1.11. Schlatter's disease (13-year-old boy – same patient as in Fig. 1.10)

Sagittal T2*: Extensive signal increase of tibial plateau apophysis. Slightly increased signal of the deep and superficial infrapatellar bursae at the posterior and anterior margins of the distal patellar tendon, consistent with reactive concomitant irritation

Fig. 1.12. Schlatter's disease (12-year-old boy)

Sagittal; *left* T1, *right* T2*: Reduced signal of distal tibial plateau apophysis on T1-weighted image and increased signal on relative T2-weighting. Initial fragmentation or defect at anterior margin (*arrows*). Slight accompanying signal changes of distal patellar tendon insertion and deep infrapatellar bursa

**Fig. 1.13. Schlatter's disease
(12-year-old girl)**

Sagittal T1: Decreased signal intensity and partial fragmentation of
tibial plateau apophysis

**Fig. 1.14. Abnormal apophyseal
ossification; small non-irritating
apophyseal ossification center of
tuberosity (38-year-old male)**

Sagittal; *left* T1, *right* T2*: Small
isolated bone fragment with fully
normal signal (*arrows*) at anterior
margin of tuberosity. Only slight
signal increase of immediately
adjacent distal patellar tendon end
in both sequences

**Fig. 1.15. Persisting apophyseal
ossification center of tuberosity.
Pronounced deep infrapatellar
bursitis (16-year-old male)**

Sagittal; *left* T1, *right* T2*: Isolated
bone fragment (*arrows*) anterior to
undulated anterior surface of tibial
plateau; closed epiphyseal cleft.
Pronounced signal decrease of
deep infrapatellar bursa (equivalent to fluid) and increased signal
intensity on relative T2-weighting
extending to adjacent posterior
margin of distal patellar tendon.
Less pronounced changes also of
superficial infrapatellar bursa

Fig. 1.16. Persisting apophyseal ossification center of tuberosity. Exudative peritendinitis (16-year-old male)

Sagittal; *left* T1, *right* T2*: Somewhat larger isolated bone fragment anterior to a bowl-shaped defect of anterior surface of tuberosity with slight thickening of distal patellar tendon and pronounced signal increase of this area in both sequences

Fig. 1.17. Persisting apophyseal ossification center/sesamoid bone in distal patellar tendon (39-year-old male)

Sagittal T1: Elongated isolated bone fragment between tuberosity and posterior margin of patellar tendon

Fig. 1.18. Persisting apophyseal ossification center at anterior margin of tibial plateau (48-year-old male)

Sagittal T1: Large roundish bone fragment between tuberosity and posterior margin of distal patellar tendon insertion

Fig. 1.19 a – c. Partial tear of distal patellar tendon with intrabursal hemorrhage – knee contusion 1 week earlier (22-year-old male)

a Sagittal; *left* T1, *right* T2*: Thickening and increased signal intensity of the distal patellar tendon, becoming more pronounced toward the tibial insertion. Fluid collection in deep infrapatellar bursa roughly triangular in configuration with upward convexity. Note bleeding-induced hyperintensity on T1-weighting and in part slightly less pronounced hyperintensity on relative T2-weighting (*arrowheads*). In addition, elongated areas of fluid signal corresponding to superficial prepatellar and infrapatellar bursae

b Sagittal T2*; **c** axial T2*: Distinct fluid level within deep infrapatellar bursa produced by settled blood components (*arrows*)

a

b

c

Fig. 1.20. Discreet partial tear of distal patellar tendon – knee contusion 10 months earlier (38-year-old female)

Sagittal; *left* T1, *right* T2*: Pronounced thickening of distal part of patellar tendon with increased signal in both sequences

Fig. 1.21. Partial tear of distal patellar tendon – contusion of tuberosity 2 months earlier (27-year-old male)

Sagittal; *left* T1, *right* T2*: Pronounced thickening of distal patellar tendon segment with increased signal intensity of posterior aspect in both sequences. In addition, mild signal reduction of adjacent anterior parts of tibial plateau on T1-weighted image (bone bruise) and local signal increase on relative T2-weighting (*arrows*)

Fig. 1.22. Exacerbated chronic tendinitis of distal patellar tendon following resection of intratendinous bone (abnormal ossification; 41-year-old female)

Sagittal; *left* T1, *right* T2*: Pronounced thickening of distal patellar tendon with increased signal intensity in both sequences; artifacts caused by metal debris at anterior margin of lesion after earlier surgical revision (*arrow*). Slightly increased fluid volume of deep infrapatellar bursa with corresponding signal increase on relative T2-weighting (*arrowhead*)

Fig. 1.23 a, b. Considerable tendinitis of distal patellar tendon; bursal edema after removal of intramedullary nail $^1/_2$ year earlier (39-year-old male)

a, b Sagittal T1: Both images show increased signal intensity and thickening of distal patellar tendon with accompanying signal decreases of adjoining subcutaneous structures, deep infrapatellar bursa, and adjacent parts of intramedullary nail drill canal. Isolated signal voids due to metal debris artifacts in the area of the old insertion site of the nail and along the course of the canal

a

b

Fig. 1.24. Tendinitis of entire patellar tendon (30-year-old male)

Sagittal T2*: Increased signal throughout the length of the patellar tendon. Hypointense margins

Fig. 1.25. Severe tendinosis/ tendinitis of patellar tendon following arthroscopy; pronounced patella baja (50-year-old female)

Sagittal; *left* T1, *right* T2*: Pronounced thickening of entire patellar tendon with considerably increased signal intensity in both sequences. In addition, slightly increased fluid volume of pre-patellar bursa with signal isointense to fluid on relative T2-weighting. Low-lying patella (Insall-Salvati ratio 0.77)

Fig. 1.26. Chronic partial tear of patellar tendon – knee contusion 11 months earlier. Tendinitis following surgical repair of rupture $^1/_2$ year earlier (68-year-old-female)

Sagittal T1: Patellar tendon show-ing thickening and buckling throughout its course, most pro-nounced proximally, with increased signal intensity on T1-weighting and circumscribed area of marrow signal at the distal end of the proximal one third, corresponding to localized calcification. Patella alta (Insall-Salvati ratio 1.29)

Fig. 1.27. Chronic partial tear of patellar tendon – knee contusion 13 years earlier (34-year-old male)

Sagittal; *left* T1, *right* T2*: In-creased signal intensity of patellar tendon throughout its course in both sequences, most pronounced in proximal portion, with partial contour disruption at inferior pole of patella (*arrows*). In addition, depiction of fluid at the posterior margin of the patellar tendon and pronounced edema of prepatellar and infrapatellar subcutaneous structures with corresponding signal increases on relatively T2-weighted image

Fig. 1.28. Very extensive partial tear of patellar tendon – knee contusion 3 weeks earlier (34-year-old male)

Sagittal; *left* T1, *right* T2*: Considerable signal increase throughout the course of the patellar tendon with marked contour incongruity in the middle third (*arrows*). Diffuse signal increase of pre-patellar/infrapatellar subcutaneous structures on relative T2-weighting caused by diffuse reactive edema. Minimal corresponding changes also within Hoffa's fat pad

Fig. 1.29. Chronic partial tear of patellar tendon – contusion $^1/_2$ year earlier (57-year-old male)

Sagittal: *left* T1, *right* T2*: V-shaped thickening of proximal patellar tendon with pronounced signal increase in both sequences. Anterior patellar insertion site elevated from inferior pole of patella. Reduced signal of anterior subcutaneous structures on T1-weighting with diffuse signal increase on relative T2-weighting, corresponding to edematous zones

Fig. 1.30. Lamellar fracture of inferior patellar pole; irritation/hemorrhage of proximal patellar tendon – trauma 1 week earlier (12-year-old boy)

Sagittal, *left* T1, *right* T2*: Mild signal decrease of inferior patellar pole on T1-weighted image. Relatively T2-weighted image showing pronounced signal increase with lamellar contour disruption basally (*arrow*). Slight thickening and increased signal of proximal half of patellar tendon. Delicate hyperintense fluid lamellae seen at posterior margin and centrally within Hoffa's fat pad on relatively T2-weighted image

Fig. 1.31. Fracture of inferior patellar pole 3 days earlier with intra- and periligamentous hemorrhage (31-year-old male)

Sagittal; *left* T1, *right* T2*: Inferior patellar pole showing reduced signal intensity on T1-weighting and increased intensity on relative T2-weighting with disruption of cortical bone and minimal posterior displacement. Area of signal increase at posterior margin of patellar tendon on relatively T2-weigthed image and increased fluid collection of pre- and infrapatellar subcutaneous structures. Delicate fluid lamellae with hyperintensity on relatively T2-weighted image also in central parts of Hoffa's fat pad

Fig. 1.32. Inferior patellar fracture 12 days earlier; intratendinous hemorrhage/partial tear of patellar tendon; partial tear of Hoffa's fat pad (55-year-old male)

Sagittal; *left* T1, *right* T2*: Inferior patellar pole showing reduced signal intensity on T1-weighted and pronounced signal increase on relatively T2-weighted image. Anterior and posterior disruptions of cortical bone. Only minimal displacement. Thickening and increased signal intensity of proximal patellar tendon segment with irregular contour near insertion. Pronounced signal decrease of prepatellar/infrapatellar subcutaneous structures on T1-weighting and pronounced signal increase on relative T2-weighting. Minimal corresponding changes of central and superoposterior parts of Hoffa's fat pad

Fig. 1.33. Inferior patellar fracture 12 days earlier; intratendinous hemorrhage/partial tear of patellar tendon; partial tear of Hoffa's fat pad; bursal hematoma (55-year-old male – same patient as in Fig. 1.32)

Sagittal; *left* T1, *right* T2*: Disrupted contour of lower patellar pole with reduced signal intensity on T1-weighted and increased signal intensity on relatively T2-weighted image. Thickening and irregularity of proximal patellar tendon with corresponding signal changes. Relatively wide midsubstance tear of fat pad, beginning anteriorly. Pronounced fluid collections in prepatellar/infrapatellar subcutaneous structures, in part involving bursal area

Fig. 1.34. Fracture of inferior patellar pole on the day before; bleeding into patellar tendon, more pronounced into prepatellar/ infrapatellar soft tissue and bursae (61-year-old female)

Sagittal; *left* T1, *right* T2*: Distinct contour disruption at inferior patellar pole with area around fracture cleft showing reduced signal intensity on T1-weighted and increased intensity on relatively T2-weighted image. No displacement. Slightly increased signal of adjacent proximal patellar tendon insertion on relatively T2-weighted image. Midsubstance tear of Hoffa's fat pad. Slightly increased signal of quadriceps tendon insertion in both sequences. Massive distention and fluid collection of prepatellar/ infrapatellar subcutaneous structures with diffusely reduced signal on T1-weighting and increased signal intensity on relatively T2-weighted image

Fig. 1.35. Fracture of inferior patellar pole 3 months earlier, profuse bleeding into patellar tendon, rather slight reaction of surrounding structures, mild tendinosis of quadriceps tendon insertion (66-year-old male)

Sagittal, *left* T1, *right* T2*: Patellar fracture cleft markedly hyperintense on relative T2-weighting; faint marginal sclerosis of absent signal intensity consistent with older trauma. Pronounced thickening of proximal patellar tendon with increased signal in both sequences. Delicate subcutaneous fluid lamellae. Posterior partial tear of fat pad. Slightly increased signal of quadriceps tendon insertion in both sequences

Fig. 1.36. Abnormal ossification of inferior patellar pole (persisting ossification center) and local irritation of tendon (15-year-old male)

Sagittal; *left* T1, *right* T2*: Normal bone marrow signal with nearly completely separated inferior patellar pole delineated by a delicate line of sclerosis. Increased signal at posterior margin of proximal patellar tendon insertion on T1-weighting and more pronounced on relative T2-weighting

Fig. 1.37. Abnormal ossification of inferior patellar pole (persisting ossification center) and local irritation of tendon (27-year-old female)

Sagittal; *left* T1, *right* T2*: Separated drop-shaped bone fragment at inferior patellar pole with fully normal bone marrow signal but circular signal increase of immediate surroundings including proximal patellar tendon attachment on relative T2-weighting

Fig. 1.38. Tendinosis of proximal patellar tendon attachment (16-year-old male)

Sagittal; *left* T1, *right* T2*: Normal bone signal. Slight V-shaped thickening of proximal patellar tendon attachment with increased signal in both sequences, most pronounced on relatively T2-weighted image (*arrows*)

Fig. 1.39. Jumper's knee; bursal and minimal osseous involvement (52-year-old male)

Sagittal; *left* T1, *right* T2*: V-shaped thickening of proximal patellar tendon with signal increase in both sequences. In addition, very discreet signal increase of anteroinferior bony attachment site on relative T2-weighting (*arrow*). Diffuse signal increase of prepatellar/infrapatellar subcutaneous structures on relatively T2-weighted image

Fig. 1.40. Pronounced jumper's knee (20-year-old male)

Sagittal; *left* T1, *right* T2*: More extensive thickening of proximal patellar tendon attachment with considerably increased signal intensity in both sequences. Slight diffuse signal increase of prepatellar/infrapatellar subcutaneous structures on relatively T2-weighted image

Fig. 1.41. Pronounced jumper's knee (17-year-old female)

Sagittal; *left* T1, *right* T2*: Considerable thickening of proximal patellar tendon with markedly increased signal intensity on T1-weighting and especially on relative T2-weighting

Fig. 1.42. Considerable jumper's knee; slight bony involvement (25-year-old male)

Sagittal; *left* T1, *right* T2*: Massive thickening of proximal patellar tendon with increased signal intensity on relative T2-weighting. Area of increased signal also extends to posterior parts of Hoffa's fat pad. Hardly discernible increase of bone signal at inferior patellar pole (*arrow*)

Fig. 1.43. Chronic local irritation following patellectomy for comminuted fracture 5 months earlier (56-year-old female)

Sagittal; *left* T1, *right* T2*: Signal void produced by metal artifact at the level of the junction of the quadriceps and patellar tendons following patellectomy. Relatively T2-weighted image showing slightly increased signal of proximal patellar tendon segments and more pronounced signal increase of anterior subcutaneous structures

Fig. 1.44 a, b. Chronic local irritation following patellectomy for comminuted fracture 1 year earlier (20-year-old female)

a Sagittal T1: Pronounced contour distention and increased signal of the quadriceps/patellar tendon junction over a length of 5 cm on T1-weighted image. Small metal artifact seen anteriorly in middle segment

b Sagittal T2*: Pronounced signal increase of the abnormal area already noted on T1-weighted image. Metal artifact in the middle segment seen more clearly

a

b

2 Quadriceps Tendon

2.1 Technique and Method

Comfortable positioning, especially of the knee, with supportive padding of the popliteal area to achieve a position in which the patient is free from pain. Axial and sagittal acquisitions using both T1- and T2-weighted sequences appear to be most useful and might be supplemented by fat-suppressed sequences as needed.

Circumscribed disorders in and around the knee should be examined using conventional extremity coils, possibly supplemented by imaging with the body coil in patients with more extensive disorders and suspected hematoma or muscle rupture.

2.2 Anatomy

The quadriceps tendon consists of a superficial portion receiving the fibers of the rectus femoris muscle and a deep portion receiving the fibers of the vastus intermedius muscle, which is joined by the tendinous fibers of the vastus medialis and vastus lateralis muscles.

The tendon fibers continue distally into the medial retinaculum and iliotibial tract as well as into the patellar tendon over the anterior surface of the patella. Most fibers of the quadriceps tendon insert into the anterior surface of the patella. The posterior insertion site is covered by synovial membrane/fat.

2.3 Normal MRI Appearance

The normal quadriceps tendon is of low signal intensity on T1- and T2-weighted images and is best seen in sagittal and axial orientations. Individual fibers can occasionally be delineated. Smooth contours.

2.4 Pathomechanism

Depending on patellar height, the quadriceps tendon moves directly over the cartilaginous or noncartilaginous part of the femoral condyles in flexion, protected from friction by synovial and subsynovial structures. The central portion of the tendon is poorly perfused.

Degenerative processes and calcifications (such as spurs at the upper margin of the patella) may contribute to partial or complete rupture of the quadriceps tendon. Quadriceps tendon tears are more frequent in males and in individuals older than 50. Bilateral tears may occur.

Quadriceps tendon ruptures tend to occur close to the patellar insertion and typically involve an indirect mechanism of injury. The tendon ruptures spontaneously or following suddenly decelerated flexion, rarely as the result of a genuine traumatic event. Predisposing conditions are gout, lupus erythematosus, diabetes, and renal failure.

Quadriceps tendon rupture is characterized by a loss of active extension and a feeling of instability when walking down stairs, occasionally leading to a fall. Some cases of ruptured tendons go unnoticed.

2.5 Pathophysiology

Tears of the quadriceps tendon are typically located close to the upper margin of the patella and may extend far toward the medial and lateral retinacula.

The extent of rupture determines whether there will be complete or partial loss of active quadriceps contraction. The former is associated with complete loss of active extension, and the patella may show slight distal displacement and anterior tilting of its upper part.

2.6 MRI Signs of Abnormal Findings

Tendinosis of Patellar Insertion

Slightly increased signal intensity of the quadriceps tendon insertion on T1- and relatively T2-weighted images without fiber discontinuity or tendon thickening (Figs. 2.1 and 2.2).

Tendon Injuries

Intratendinous signal intensity increases with the severity of the injury in all sequences. Damage may range from various degrees of disruption of individual fiber bundles to complete disruption of fiber continuity with retraction of the free ends (Figs. 2.3–2.7).

The severity of injury also determines the extent of bleeding into surrounding structures, as indicated on MRI by increased signal intensities, predominantly on relative and pure T2-weighting. Organized hematomas developing after partial tears or scar formation may be identified as areas of lower signal intensity (Figs. 2.8 and 2.9).

2.7 Clinical Role of MRI Findings

Rupture of the quadriceps tendon is diagnosed clinically. The degree of loss of active extension correlates with the extent of the lesion (partial or complete tendon tear, tendon tear with involvement of retinaculum). Interpretation of the MRI findings should concentrate on the extent of rupture.

Surgical exploration of the quadriceps tendon must always include the full length of the tendon, irrespective of the MRI findings. Healing of chronic quadriceps tendon tears may be associated with elongation of the tendon due to scar formation. The extent of elongation can be estimated by comparing the distance from the muscle belly to the upper patellar margin with the contralateral side.

Further Reading

Calvo E, Ferrer A, Robledo AG, Alvarez L, Castill F, Vallejo C (1997) Bilateral simultaneous spontaneous quadriceps tendons rupture. A case report studied by magnetic resonance imaging. Clin Imaging 21 (1): 73–76

Insall J, Salvati E (1971) Patellar position in the normal knee. Radiology 101: 101–104

Petersen W et al. (1999) Blutgefäßversorgung der Quadrizepssehne. Unfallchirurg 102: 543–547

Pomeranz SJ (1977) Gamuts and pearls in MRI and orthopedics. MRI-EFI Publications, pp 191–192

Schweitzer ME, Mitchell DG, Ehrlich SM (1993) The patellar tendon: thickening, internal signal buckling, and other MR variants. Skeletal Radiol 22 (6): 411–416

Spector ED, Di Marcangelo MT, Jacoby JH (1995) The radiologic diagnosis of quadriceps tendon rupture. N J Med 92 (9): 590–592

Table 2.1. Characteristic signal intensities

	T1w	T2w	T2*w	rho-w	FAT-SAT
Tendons	0	0	0 – ↑	0	0
Fatty tissue	↑↑	↑	0 – ↑	↑↑	0
Compact/spongy bone	0	0	0	0	0
Marrow (yellow)	↑↑↑	↑ – ↑↑	0 – ↑	↑↑	0
Muscle tissue	↑	↑	↑	↑↑	↑
Effusion (serous)	↑ – 0	↑↑↑	↑↑↑	↑ – ↑↑	↑↑↑
Hemarthrosis	↑↑	↑↑	↑↑	↑↑↑	↑↑

0 No signal; ↑ low SI; ↑↑ intermediate SI; ↑↑↑ high SI.

Fig. 2.1. Mild tendinosis of quadriceps tendon insertion (36-year-old male)

Sagittal; *left* T1, *right* T2*: Slightly increased signal intensity of the quadriceps tendon insertion at the upper pole of the patella in both sequences; patella alta (Insall-Salvati ratio 1.45)

Fig. 2.2. Extensive tendinosis of quadriceps tendon insertion (16-year-old female)

Sagittal; *left* T1, *right* T2*: Marked increase in signal intensity of the anterior quadriceps tendon insertion, especially on relatively T2-weighted image (*arrow*)

Fig. 2.3. Partial tear of quadriceps tendon – knee contusion on the day before (21-year-old male)

Sagittal; *left* T1, *right* T2*: Thickening and irregular contour of distal portion of quadriceps tendon with pronounced signal increase on relatively T2-weighted image. Dense area within Hoffa's fat pad (*right image*) due to boundary artifacts/fibrosis

Fig. 2.4 a, b. Very extensive, almost subtotal partial tear of quadriceps tendon – dashboard injury 6 weeks earlier (33-year-old female)

a Sagittal T1: Pronounced thickening of distal segment of quadriceps tendon with increased signal intensity – extent of discontinuity appreciated more clearly on T2*-weighted image

b Sagittal T2*: Pronounced signal increase of the segment already abnormal on the T1-weighted image with discontinuity of the distal half of the tendon near its anterior insertion and edema/hemorrhage of adjoining tendon parts

a

b

Fig. 2.5. Partial degenerative tear of quadriceps tendon with slight bony involvement (46-year-old male)

Sagittal; *left* T1, *right* T2*: Elongated area of increased signal intensity of thickened distal quadriceps tendon segment with distention of isolated fibers and small lamellar bony contour elevation at anterior upper pole of patella

Fig. 2.6. (Subtotal) tear of quadriceps tendon insertion – trauma 2 weeks earlier; patellar tendinitis; bleeding into prepatellar soft tissue (46-year-old male)

Sagittal; *left* T1, *right* T2*: Massive thickening of distal quadriceps tendon with fluid signal. Only inadequate, tube-like residual fibers in the posterior margin of the tendon with complete discontinuity of the bulk of the tendon anteriorly. Relatively T2-weighted image shows fluid collections of high signal intensity extending into prepatellar area. Proximal half of patellar tendon also shows slightly increased signal intensity but without disruption of continuity

a

b

c

d

Fig. 2.7a–d. Complete quadriceps tendon rupture on the day before (60-year-old male)

a Sagittal T1: Considerable contour distention and reduced signal in the area of the former quadriceps tendon insertion

b Axial T2*: Diffusely increased signal of the irregular residual fibers of quadriceps tendon in the area of rupture. Sickle-shaped fluid collections in anterior subcutaneous structures and pronounced joint effusion

c, d Sagittal T2*: Extent of tendinous contour disruptions at the superior patellar pole discerned much more clearly due to fluid signal intensity of the area including subcutaneous fluid lamellae and joint effusion

Fig. 2.8. Chronic, partly organized hematoma of anterior distal quadriceps tendon following quadriceps contusion/partial tear – traumatic suprapatellar impact $1/_2$ year earlier (40-year-old male)

Sagittal; *left* T1, *right* T2*: Both sequences show ovoid thickening and increased signal intensity of anterior aspect of tendon-muscle junction and intact, well-defined contours. Diffuse reactive edema of prepatellar subcutaneous tissue

Fig. 2.9. Fibrosis of quadriceps tendon insertion as a late sequela of trauma – contusion 8 years earlier (25-year-old male)

Sagittal T1: Hypointense thickening of distal quadriceps tendon but fairly regular contours (no signal increase on relative T2-weighting – *not shown*)

3 Anterior Cruciate Ligament

3.1 Technique and Method

The knee should be positioned with 10°–15° of external rotation to bring the anterior cruciate ligament (ACL) into the sagittal plane. Alternatively, the same effect can be achieved by tilting of the imaging plane (sagittal oblique orientation). Specific queries regarding the area of the ACL may require a slice thickness of 3 mm. Sagittal (oblique), coronal, and axial imaging planes.

Sagittal sections provide the best overview while coronal and axial projections may yield useful additional information, especially in inconclusive cases. Also helpful are 3D acquisitions with reconstruction of the area of interest and direct 3D visualization of the ACL (higher spatial resolution but poorer image contrast).

3.2 Anatomy

The ACL is a 3–4 cm long band of parallel fibers that extends from the medial side of the anterior tibial plateau to the most posterior aspect of the medial surface of the lateral femoral condyle. Anatomic measurements have shown that the center of the tibial attachment is situated at 41–43% of the greatest sagittal diameter of the tibial plateau (0% anteriorly, 100% posteriorly); see Diagram 1a, p. 59.

Using the quadrant method according to Bernard and Hertel (1996), the center of the femoral attachment of the ACL as seen from the side lies in the distal lower corner of the uppermost posterior quadrant, which is at 25% of the greatest posterior condyle diameter measured along Blumensaat's line (0% posteriorly, 100% anteriorly) and at 25% of the height of the femoral condyle measured perpendicular to this line (0% superiorly, 100% inferiorly); see Diagram 1b, p. 59.

The diameter of the ACL is smaller in its midportion than at its attachments (trumpet-shaped configuration). The course of the ACL is straight in nearly full knee extension and slightly curved when the joint is flexed. In extension, its anterior fibers run parallel to Blumensaat's line.

Hyperlaxity of the knee joint may be associated with physiologic diversion of the anterior ACL fibers around the anterior edge of the intercondylar notch. Depending on the extension and configuration of the infrapatellar plica (mucous ligament), there is variable covering of the ACL by synovium or structures of the plica.

3.3 Normal MRI Appearance

Well-defined contour, straight course, delineation of individual fiber bundles. Mainly of intermediate signal intensity when the fibers are fanned, decreasing intensity with more compact bundling of fibers. High-signal-intensity areas correspond to synovium and/or fatty tissue (Figs. 3.1–3.5).

3.4 Pathomechanism

The ACL can undergo partial or complete rupture, either alone or in conjunction with injury to other ligaments of the knee.

Isolated ACL rupture is most commonly caused by extension/hyperextension with internal rotation as well as deceleration during active quadriceps muscle contraction.

Combined injuries are induced by excessive flexing rotation (e.g. "unhappy triad" comprising injury of ACL, medial collateral ligament, and medial meniscus), by flexion/external rotation/abduction, by opening mechanisms, and by pronounced translation.

3.5 Pathophysiology

Cruciate ligament injuries are associated with hemarthrosis in 80–90% of cases. Concomitant injuries are likely, involving in particular the medial collateral ligament, both menisci, the cartilage and subchondral bone (bone bruises) of the posterior tibial plateau (anterior tibial subluxation), the anterior femoral condyle (hyperextension mechanism), and the bony capsular attachments (avulsions of anterolateral tibial plateau – Segond fragment, posteromedial or posterolateral edge of tibial plateau). When the synovial sheath remains intact, ACL rupture may be anatomically incomplete but still result in complete loss of function.

3.6 MRI Signs of Abnormal Findings

- Intraligamentous signal changes (focal or generalized).
- Internal structural irregularities (spreading and undulation of fibers, blurring, partial disruption).
- Changes in diameter (focal or generalized thickening/thinning).
- Changes in external contour (well-defined, irregular, partial or complete contour disruption).
- Changes in course (abnormal curving, kinking, flattening; abnormal (horizontal) orientation, retraction).
- Paraligamentous changes: bleeding/effusion into synovial sheath, synovial thickening, ovoid pseudomass (may be seen on coronal sections as double-eye sign), octopus sign (tentacle-like remnants of ligament/vessels after complete rupture).
- Bony avulsion of femoral or tibial ligament insertion (Figs. 3.17 and 3.18).
- Femorotibial malalignment (anterior subluxation of tibia relative to femoral condyles).

Constellation of Findings Suggesting ACL Injury

Bone bruises of posterolateral tibial plateau, perhaps also of anterior aspect of lateral femoral condyle (hypointense microfracture zones on T1-weighted images and increased signal on relative T2-weighting): correlated with ACL tear in 87% of cases (valgus stress/hyperextension/subluxation).

There are often concomitant injuries of the medial collateral ligament and rupture of the medial/lateral meniscus (unhappy triad). Secondary hemarthrosis. Effusion less pronounced or developing later in cruciate ligament injury without bone involvement.

3.7 MRI Grading of ACL Injuries

Based on the widely accepted international classification of ligament injuries of the American Medical Association, the following grades of ligament injuries are distinguished on MRI:

I. Strain/Subtle Midsubstance Tear

Only intraligamentous structural changes. Increased signal intensity on T1- and T2*-weighted images, bulk of fibers intact, and unimpaired external configuration (unchanged contour, thickness, length; Figs. 3.6 and 3.7).

II. Partial Tear

Increased signal intensity in both sequences and thickening (intraligamentous edema/hemorrhage, possibly pseudomass), contour and fiber irregularities or partial discontinuity (Figs. 3.8–3.10).

III. Complete Tear

Pronounced increase in signal intensity, discontinuity, potential retraction, deviation from normal course, possibly pseudomass (Figs. 3.11–3.16).

3.8 MRI Pitfalls in ACL Injury

- Oblique sectioning of posterior femoral cortex (with black bone contour mimicking intact femoral ACL insertion) – to avoid this pitfall, comparison with coronal and axial slices in inconclusive cases and, if needed, also additional slices (thin-section images, readjusted section orientation).
- Altogether poor visualization of femoral ACL portion, depending on positioning of the knee/ angulation of sagittal sections.
- Intrasynovial bleeding may make rupture grading difficult or inaccurate.
- High fat content of cruciate ligament may mimic bleeding in very rare cases.
- Fibrosis associated with chronic tears may mimic an intact ligament as scar tissue is hypointense on T1- and T2-weighted images (Fig. 3.21).
- Aplasia of cruciate ligament.

3.9 Clinical Role of MRI Findings

The MRI diagnosis of ACL rupture must be interpreted in conjunction with the overall clinical assessment.

Crucial factors are a history of prior injury, reconstruction of the mechanism of injury, and analysis of subjective and objective instability. Objective instability is most reliably determined by the drawer test in near extension (Lachman test) or by examination under anesthesia.

Most MRI grade I and II cruciate ligament tears can be treated conservatively since some of these ligament injuries heal spontaneously. The indication for surgery in grade III tears is determined by the degree of subjective instability and the individual patient's needs.

Management of concomitant injuries may in some cases have priority over treating ACL injuries (meniscal displacement, osteochondral fragments, defined avulsions of collateral ligament insertions).

Further Reading

American Medical Association Commitee on the Medical Aspects of Sport (1968) Standard Nomenclature of Athletics Injuries. American Medical Association, Chicago

Barry KP, Mesgarzadeh M, Triolo J, Moyer R, Tehranzadeh J, Bonakdarpour A (1996) Accuracy of MRI patterns in evaluating anterior cruciate ligament tears. Skeletal Radiol 25 (4): 365–370

Bernard M, Hertel P, Hornung H, Cierpinski T (1997) Femoral insertion of the ACL-radiographic quadrant method. Am J Knee Surg 10: 14–22

Boisgard S, Levai JP, Geiger B, Saidane K, Landjerit B (1999) Study of the variations in length of the anterior cruciate ligament during flexion of the knee: use of a 3D model reconstructed from MRI sections. Surg Radiol Anat 21 (5): 313–317

Table 3.1. Characteristic signal intensities

	T1w	T2w	T2*w	rho-w	FAT-SAT
ACL					
Collagen fiber bundles	0	0	0 – ↑	0	0
Synovium	↑	↑↑	↑↑	↑↑	0
Fresh hemorrhage	0 – ↑	↑↑	↑↑	↑↑	↑
Bone bruise	0 – ↑	↑	↑↑ – ↑↑↑	↑ – ↑↑	↑↑ – ↑↑↑
Intraligamentous edema	↑	↑ – ↑↑	↑↑ – ↑↑↑	↑	↑↑↑
Ligament tear	↑ – ↑↑	↑↑ – ↑↑↑	↑↑ – ↑↑↑	↑↑	↑↑↑

0 No signal; ↑ low SI; ↑↑ intermediate SI; ↑↑↑ high SI.

Dimond PM, Fadale PD, Hulstyn MJ, Tung GA, Greisberg J (1998) A comparison of MRI findings in patients with acute and chronic ACL tears. Am J Knee Surg 11 (3): 153–159

Do Dai DD, Youngberg RA, Lanchbury FD, Pitcher JD, Garver TH (1996) Intraligamentous ganglion cysts of the anterior cruciate ligament: MR findings with clinical and arthroscopic correlations. J Comput Assist Tomogr 20 (1): 80–84

Faber J et al. (1999) Occult osteochondral lesions after anterior curciate ligament rupture, six-year magnetic resonance imaging follow up-study. Am J Sports Med 27: 489–494

Friedman RL, Jackson DW (1996) Magnetic resonance imaging of the anterior cruciate ligament: current concepts. Orthopedics 19 (6): 525–532

Ho CP, Marks PH, Steadman JR (1999) MR imaging of knee anterior cruciate ligament and associated injuries in skiers. Magn Reson Imaging Clin N Am 7 (1): 117–130

Jee WH, Choe BY, Kim JM, Song HH; Choi KH (1998) MRT des Kniegelenkes: Fehleranalyse bezüglich der Meniskus- und Kreuzbanddiagnostik an einem arthroskopisch kontrollierten Patientenkollektiv. Rofo Fortschr Geb Röntgenstr Neuen Bildgeb Verfahr 169 (2): 157–162

Kuhne JH, Durr HR, Steinborn M, Jansson V, Refior HJ (1998) Magnetic resonance imaging and knee stability following ACL reconstruction. Orthopedics 21 (1): 39–43

Lawrance JA, Ostlere SJ, Dodd CA (1996) MRI diagnosis of partial tears of the anterior cruciate ligament. Injury 27 (3): 153–155

Lee K, Siegel MJ, Lau DM, Hildebolt CF, Matava MJ (1999) Anterior cruciate ligament tears: MR imaging-based diagnosis in a pediatric population. Radiology 213 (3): 697–704

Lindner DM Kamaric E, Moseley JB, Noble PC (1995) Partial tears of the anterior cruciate ligament. Are they clinically detectable. Am J Sports Med 23: 111

McCauley TR, Moses M, Kier R, Lynch JK, Barton JW, Jokl P (1994) MR diagnosis of tears of anterior cruciate ligament of the knee: importance of ancillary findings. AJR Am J Roentgenol 162 (1): 115–119

Mc Dermott MJ, Bathgate B, Gillingham BL, Hennrikus WL (1998) Correlation of MRI and arthroscopic diagnosis of knee pathology in children and adolescents. J Pediatr Orthop 18 (5): 675–678

Munk B, Madsen F, Lundorf E, Staunstrup H, Schmidt SA, Bolvig L, Hellfritzsch MB, Jensen J (1998) Clinical magnetic resonance imaging and arthroscopic findings in knees: a comparative prospective study of meniscus anterior cruciate ligament and cartilage lesions. Arthroscopy 14 (2): 171–175

Murao H, Morishita S, Nakajima M, Abe M (1998) Magnetic resonance imaging of anterior cruciate ligament (ACL) tears: diagnostic value of ACL-tibial plateau angle. J Orthop Sci 3 (1): 10–17

Niitsu M, Ikeda K, Itai Y (1998) Slightly flexed knee position within a standard knee coil: MR delineation of the anterior cruciate ligament. Eur Radiol 8 (1): 113–115

Pomeranz SJ (1991) Orthopaedic MR. JB Lippincott, Philadelphia, S 131

Quinn SF, Brown TR, Demlow TA (1993) MR diagnosis of tears of anterior cruciate ligament of the knee: importance of ancillary findings. J Magn Reson Imaging 3 (6): 843–847

Rappeport ED, Wieslander SB, Stephensen S, Lausten GS, Thomsen HS (1997) MRI preferable to diagnostic arthroscopy in knee joint injuries. A double-blind comparison of 47 patients. Acta Orthop Scand 68 (3): 277–281

Riel KA, Reinisch M, Kersting Sommerhoff B, Hof N, Merl T (1999) 0.2-Tesla magnetic resonance imaging of internal lesions of the knee joint: a prospective arthroscopically controlled clinical study. Knee Surg Sports Traumatol Arthrosc 7 (1): 37–41

Roychowdhury S, Fitzgerald SW, Sonin AH, Peduto AJ, Miller FH, Hoff Fl (1997) Using MR imaging to diagnose partial tears of the anterior cruciate ligament: value of axial images. AJR Am J Roentgenol 168 (6): 1487–1491

Schaefer WD, Martin DF, Pope TL Jr, Rudicil HS (1996) Meniscal ossicle. J South Orthop Assoc 5 (2): 126–129

Shelbourne KD, Jennings RW, Vahey TN (1999) Magnetic resonance imaging of posterior cruciate ligament injuries: assessment of healing. Am J Knee Surg 12 (4): 209–213

Smith DK, May DA, Phillips P (1996) MR imaging of the anterior cruciate ligament: frequency of discordant findings on sagittal-oblique images and correlation with arthroscopic findings. AJR Am J Roentgenol 166 (2): 411–413

Stäubli HU, Adam O, Becker W, Burgkart R (1999) Anterior cruciate ligament and intercondylar notch in the coronal oblique plane: anatomy complemented by magnetic resonance imaging in cruciate ligament-intact knees. Arthroscopy 15 (4): 349–359

Stäubli HU, Rauschning W (1994) Tibial attachment area of the anterior cruciate ligament in the extended knee position. Knee Surg Sports Traumatol Arthrosc 2: 138–146

Uppal A, Disler DG, Short WB, Mc Cauley TR, Cooper JA (1998) Internal derangements of the knee: rates of occurrence at MR imaging in patients referred by orthopedic surgeons compared with rates in patients referred by physicians who are not orthopedic surgeons. Radiology 207 (3): 633–636

**Fig. 3.1. Normal ACL
(35-year-old male)**

Sagittal T1: Normal course of
ligament; compact fibers of low
signal intensity. Fibers parallel to
Blumensaat's line

**Fig. 3.2. Normal ACL
(35-year-old male)**

Sagittal T2*: Normal course of
ligament; compact fibers of low
signal intensity

**Fig. 3.3. Normal ACL
(19-year-old female)**

Sagittal T1: Normal course of
ligament with femoral portion
lying out of slice

**Fig. 3.4. Normal ACL
(14-year-old girl)**

Sagittal; *left* T1, *right* T2*: Normal
course of ligament with smooth,
slightly fanned fibers; low signal
intensity in anterior portion and
intermediate intensity in posterior
portion

**Fig. 3.5. Normal ACL
(36-year-old male)**

Sagittal; *left* T1, *right* T2*: Normal
course of ligament with smooth,
slightly fanned fibers; intermediate
signal intensity

**Fig. 3.6. ACL strain – grade I
lesion (26-year-old male)**

Sagittal; *left* T1, *right* T2*: Both
sequences show increased signal
intensity of ACL, more pronounced
in tibial two thirds, slight spreading
of fibers, bulk of fibers intact

Fig. 3.7. Strain/subtle intrasubstance tear of ACL 6 days earlier – grade I lesion (9-year-old girl)

Sagittal; *left* T1, *right* T2*: Increased signal intensity of ACL in both sequences with intraligamentous edema and spreading of fibers; main continuity still intact as seen in particular on relative T2-weighting (*right image*)

Fig. 3.8. Partial ACL tear, femoral portion, grade II – distortion 1 week earlier (35-year-old female)

Sagittal; *left* T1, *right* T2*: Increased signal intensity of ACL in both sequences with spreading of fibers; irregularity and partial discontinuity near femoral insertion (*arrows*) but main fibers still continuous. Reactive effusion

Fig. 3.9. Partial ACL tear, grade II (24-year-old male)

Sagittal; *left* T1, *right* T2*: Increased signal intensity of ACL in both sequences with spreading of fibers and intraligamentous edema; discreet partial discontinuity. Fluid extension into clefts of Hoffa's fat pad. Reactive effusion

Fig. 3.10. Partial ACL tear, grade II – 6-week history of increasing instability without known trauma (53-year-old male)

Sagittal; *left* T1, *right* T2*: Pronounced signal increase of ACL in both sequences with marked thickening and spreading of fibers. Relative T2-weighting shows partial continuity of fibers (*right image*)

Fig. 3.11. (Subtotal) ACL tear, femoral portion, grade II – III, 2 days earlier – surgery: complete rupture (16-year-old male)

Sagittal; *left* T1, *right* T2*: Massive thickening of femoral half of ACL, abnormal signal increase in both sequences, insufficient residual continuity (*arrows*)

Fig. 3.12. (Subtotal) ACL tear, grade II – III, 2 days earlier – surgery: grade III lesion (29-year-old male)

Sagittal; *left* T1, *right* T2*: Thickening of ACL throughout its course with increased signal intensity in both sequences – considerable irregularities of central half/ proximal third, some fibers with insufficient residual continuity in posterior portion

Fig. 3.13 a, b. ACL tear, grade III, 4 days earlier (15-year-old female)

a Sagittal T1: Highly irregular course of ligament; adequate fiber continuity not discernible, especially in proximal and central portions. Abnormal course with slight posterior convexity

b Sagittal T2*: Clear depiction of extent of damage of proximal/central portion (*arrow*)

a

b

Fig. 3.14. Fresh ACL tear, grade III, central third – injury on the day before (36-year-old male)

Sagittal; *left* T1, *right* T2*: Completely irregular course of fibers with a defect zone in the central third of the ligament. T1-weighting shows a hyperintense focal intraligamentous hemorrhage in this zone (*arrow*). Posterior defect of Hoffa's fat pad. Straining of capsule. Hemarthrosis

Fig. 3.15. ACL tear, grade III, 2 weeks earlier (22-year-old male)

Sagittal; *left* T1, *right* T2*: Destruction of proximal half of ligament with some irregular, partly tentacle-like, residual fibers (faint octopus sign). Tibial retraction of ligament, abnormal course. Hemarthrosis

Fig. 3.16. ACL tear, grade III (15-year-old female)

Sagittal; *left* T1, *right* T2*: Nonvisualization of ACL with diffuse, netlike structures replacing femoral two thirds. Posterior cruciate ligament showing slightly increased signal intensity in proximal portion due to straining but no discontinuity. Reactive effusion

Fig. 3.17. Bony avulsion of tibial ACL insertion, tibial plateau fracture 2 weeks earlier (42-year-old female)

Sagittal; *left* T1, *right* T2*: Tibial ACL insertion with bony discontinuity and elevation of a bony lamella into the joint space. Adjacent tibial fracture lines/marrow edema. Pronounced signal increase of tibial two thirds of ACL – functional grade III ligament tear. Considerable reactive effusion. Distal patellar tendinosis. Edema of anterior soft tissue structures

a

b

c

d

Fig. 3.18 a – d. Eminence avulsion 3 weeks earlier (48-year-old male)

a Sagittal T1: Straight to curved fracture line through tibial plateau, partly at the level of the former epiphyseal cleft, extending to the anterior margin of the ACL insertion and to the base of posterior cruciate ligament. No displacement. ACL intact with just slightly increased signal intensity in posterior aspect

b Sagittal T2*: Hyperintensity of tibial plateau fracture line and of ACL, especially in posterior portions. Intact fibers in anterior part. Slight joint effusion

c Coronal T1: Curvilinear signal decrease showing the course of the fracture line through the base of eminence. No displacement

d Axial T2*: Fragment of eminence demarcated by hyperintense margin (*arrows*)

Fig. 3.19. Old (subtotal) ACL tear, grade III, 13 years earlier/posttraumatic atrophy (31-year-old female)

Sagittal T1: Thin residual ACL structures taking an abnormal course with posterior convexity

Fig. 3.20 a, b. Old ACL tear, 1 $\frac{1}{4}$ years earlier – old grade III lesion (30-year-old male)

a Sagittal T1: Nonvisualization of proximal two thirds of ACL. Irregular linear residual structures. No reactive effusion

b Coronal T1: Typical vertical ligament structures absent at medial margin of lateral condyle (*arrow*). Irregular residual structure superiorly – cf. normal appearance in Fig. 4.1

a

b

Fig. 3.21. Fibrosis of ACL after partial tear 15 years earlier – old grade II lesion (55-year-old male)

Sagittal; *left* T1, *right* T2*: Abnormally curved course of a very thin and conspicuously hypointense ACL. Slight reactive effusion. Prepatellar/infrapatellar soft tissue edema

Fig. 3.22. ACL repair 3 years earlier, intact suture (42-year-old male)

Sagittal; *left* T1, *right* T2*: Normal course of only slightly thinned ACL with isolated small signal voids along the course of the ligament due to metal artifacts, most clearly seen on relative T2-weighting (*right image*)

4 Posterior Cruciate Ligament

4.1 Technique and Method

The posterior cruciate ligament can be examined using axial, coronal, and sagittal T1- and T2-weighted sequences. Comfortable positioning in an extremity coil. The slice thickness should be 4 mm or less.

4.2 Anatomy

The posterior cruciate ligament (PCL) is the strongest ligament of the knee. It courses from the anterolateral surface of the medial femoral condyle (cartilage-bone junction) to the most posterior, sloping part of the tibial insertion area.

The PCL extends in a fan-shaped manner and, functionally, can be subdivided into an anterolateral and a posteromedial part. Anatomically, however, these two parts are not clearly distinct from one another.

Stabilizing meniscofemoral ligaments course from the femoral condyle to the posterior horn of the lateral meniscus, passing the PCL anteriorly and posteriorly (ligaments of Humphry and Wrisberg, respectively).

4.3 Normal MRI Appearance

The PCL appears as a well-defined, homogeneous black band on T1- and T2-weighted images and is present on at least two consecutive scans obtained in sagittal orientation. Since the PCL is relaxed when the knee is extended, its course is frequently seen as slightly curved.

Humphry's ligament (anterior) and Wrisberg's ligament (posterior) are depicted on sagittal sections as small circular structures of no signal in the immediate vicinity of the PCL (Figs. 4.1 and 4.2).

4.4 Pathomechanism/Pathophysiology

The PCL is most frequently injured through antero-posterior translation of the tibial plateau with the knee flexed. This is why this mechanism of injury is frequently associated with contusion (bone bruises) of the anterior tibial plateau. Additional external rotation components of the lower leg make PCL injury more likely.

Combined injuries are caused by more pronounced displacement in this position or by opening mechanisms (varus-valgus injuries). Rupture of the PCL and the respective collateral ligament in this constellation may be associated with additional ACL rupture.

4.5 MRI Signs of Abnormal Findings

- Intraligamentous signal increases (focal or generalized).
- Internal structural irregularities (spreading and undulation of fibers, blurring, partial disruption).
- Changes in diameter (focal or generalized thickening/thinning).
- Changes in external contour (irregular, partial or complete contour disruption – while synovial sheath may be intact).
- Changes in course (more pronounced curving; kinking and retraction rare).
- Paraligamentous changes: bleeding/effusion into synovial sheath, synovial thickening, pseudo-mass.
- Bony avulsions, predominantly of tibial insertion (Figs. 4.16 – 4.19).
- Femorotibial malalignment (anterior displacement/subluxation of femur relative to tibia – to a lesser degree also present with ligamental hyperelasticity, insufficiency, or laxity).

The PCL requires a violent force to rupture. PCL rupture may be accompanied by injury to the following structures: medial collateral ligament (50%), ACL (65%), medial meniscus (33%), lateral collateral ligament/capsular area (10%).

4.6 MRI Grading of PCL Injuries

Based on the widely accepted international classification of ligament injuries of the American Medical Association, the following grades of ligament injuries are distinguished on MRI:

I. Strain/Subtle Midsubstance Tear

Only intraligamentous structural changes. Increased signal intensity on T1- and T2*-weighted images, bulk of fibers intact, and unimpaired external configuration (unchanged contour, thickness, length; Figs. 4.3–4.5).

II. Partial Tear

Increased signal intensity on T1- and relatively T2-weighted images with thickening (intraligamentous edema/hemorrhage, possibly pseudomass), contour and fiber irregularities or partial discontinuity (Figs. 4.6–4.10).

III. Complete Tear

Pronounced increase in signal intensity, thickening, (central) discontinuity, retraction less common compared to ACL because of thicker synovial sheath, abnormal course, possibly pseudomass (Figs. 4.11–4.15).

4.7 MRI Pitfalls in PCL Injury

- Acute bleeding along the course of the ligament (masking of ligament structures – caveat: inaccurate assessment of severity of injury).
- No retraction of free ends when the synovial sheath is intact despite complete PCL rupture (underestimation of grade).
- Masking of the PCL by inflammatory synovial processes.

Note: Because of the deep tibial insertion of the PCL 1 cm below the joint plateau, arthroscopy may fail to detect distal tears unless posterior or intercondylar portals, hook probes, and shavers are used.

4.8 Clinical Role of MRI Findings

In patients with complex injuries requiring acute management of PCL injury, MRI provides crucial information on the location of the PCL injury (proximal, distal) and for selecting the surgical access (anterior or posterior).

The degree of instability determines whether repair or replacement of the PCL is indicated. Instability is most reliably determined by stress radiographs or instrumented measurement in 90° of knee flexion with comparison to the contralateral side. MRI provides no information on stability.

Table 4.1. Characteristic signal intensities

	T1w	T2w	T2*w	rho-w	FAT-SAT
PCL	0	0	0 – ↑	0	0
Partial tear	↑ – ↑↑	↑↑	↑↑	↑	↑↑
Complete tear	↑ – ↑↑	↑↑↑	↑↑ – ↑↑↑	↑↑	↑↑↑

0 No signal; ↑ low SI; ↑↑ intermediate SI; ↑↑↑ high SI.

Further Reading

Jee WH, Choe BY, Kim JM, Song HH, Choi KH (1998) MRT des Kniegelenkes: Fehleranalyse bezüglich der Meniskus- und Kreuzbanddiagnostik an einem arthroskopisch kontrollierten Patientenkollektiv. Rofo Fortschr Geb Röntgenstr Neuen Bildgeb Verfahr 169 (2): 157–162

McDermott MJ, Bathgate B, Gillingham BL, Hennrikus WL (1998) Correlation of MRI and arthroscopic diagnosis of knee pathology in children and adolescents. J Pediatr Orthop 18 (5): 675–678

Patten RM, Richardson ML, Zink Brody G, Rolfe BA (1994) Complete vs. partial-thickness tears of the posterior cruciate ligament: MR findings. J Comput Assist Tomogr 18 (5): 793–799

Rappeport ED, Wieslander SB, Stephensen S, Lausten GS, Thomsen HS (1997) MRI preferable to diagnostic arthroscopy in knee joint injuries. A double-blind comparison of 47 patients. Acta Orthop Scand 68 (3): 277–281

Riel KA, Reinisch M, Kersting Sommerhoff B, Hof N, Merl T (1999) 0.2-Tesla magnetic resonance imaging of internal lesions of the knee joint: a prospective arthroscopically controlled clinical study. Knee Surg Sports Traumatol Arthrosc 7 (1): 37–41

Shelbourne KD, Jennings RW, Vahey TN (1999) Magnetic resonance imaging of posterior cruciate ligament injuries: assessment of healing. Am J Knee Surg 12 (4): 209–213

Sonin AH, Fitzgerald SW, Friedman H, Hoff FL, Hendrix RW, Rogers LF (1994) Posterior cruciate ligament injury: MR imaging diagnosis and patterns of injury. Radiology 190 (2): 455–458

Tewes DP, Fritts HM, Fields RD, Quick DC, Buss DD (1997) Chronically injured posterior cruciate ligament: magnetic resonance imaging. Clin Orthop 335: 224–232

Uppal A, Disler DG, Short WB, McCauley TR, Cooper JA (1998) Internal derangements of the knee: rates of occurrence at MR imaging in patients referred by orthopedic surgeons compared with rates in patients referred by physicians who are not orthopedic surgeons. Radiology 207 (3): 633–636

**Fig. 4.1. Normal PCL
(53-year-old female)**

Coronal T1: PCL depicted as a
roundish hypointense structure
at the lateral margin of the medial
condyle (*arrow*). ACL visualized
as a vertically oriented, slightly
curved linear structure at the
medial margin of the lateral
condyle (*arrowhead*)

**Fig. 4.2. Normal PCL
(25-year-old male)**

Sagittal T1: Hypointense band with
slightly curved proximal portion
between posterior margin of intercondylar notch and posterior tibial
plateau

Fig. 4.3 a, b. Strain/discreet intrasubstance tear of PCL, 1 year earlier and again 1 month earlier (42-year-old male)

a Sagittal T1: High-signal-intensity zone in the midportion of the PCL (*arrow*)

b Sagittal T2*: Pronounced signal increase also on relatively T2-weighted image

Fig. 4.4. Strain/discreet partial tear of proximal PCL, 3 months earlier, grade I lesion; slight joint effusion (31-year-old male)

Sagittal; *left* T1, *right* T2*: Increased signal intensity of proximal third of PCL, especially on relatively T2-weighted image, with slight thickening near insertion but intact main continuity. Slight joint effusion

Fig. 4.5 a, b. Partial PCL tear, grade I, 6 weeks earlier (31-year-old male)

a Sagittal T1: Increased signal intensity of central/distal PCL

b Sagittal T2*: Signal increase much more pronounced than on T1-weighting, especially in the central third of the PCL

a

b

Fig. 4.6 a, b. Partial PCL tear, grade I – II – long history of recurrent posterior knee pain without traumatic event (36-year-old male)

a Sagittal T1; **b** sagittal T2*: Marked central hyperintensity throughout the course of the PCL in both sequences. Tube- to rail-like marginal continuity. Slight joint effusion

Fig. 4.7. (Subtotal) PCL tear, grade (II –) III – knee contusion/distortion 4 weeks earlier (18-year-old male)

Sagittal T1: Marked hyperintensity of distal three quarters of PCL. Almost complete disruption of posterior contour in distal third (*arrow*)

Fig. 4.8 a, b. (Subtotal) PCL tear, grade (II –) III – knee contusion 1 week earlier (39-year-old male)

a Sagittal T1: Increased signal intensity and contour distension of PCL, most pronounced in central third – inadequate residual continuity

b Sagittal T2*: Extent of injury seen even more clearly

a

b

Fig. 4.9. (Subtotal) PCL rupture, grade (II –) III – knee contusion 2 weeks earlier (25-year-old male)

Sagittal; *left* T1, *right* T2*: Considerable contour distension and signal increase of PCL throughout its course, most pronounced in the central third with focal contour disruptions

**Fig. 4.10. PCL tear, grade III –
knee distortion 2 weeks earlier
(16-year-old male)**

Sagittal; *left* T1, *right* T2*: Increased signal intensity of PCL in
posterior two thirds with contour
distention and nearly complete
discontinuity of middle portion

**Fig. 4.11. PCL tear, grade III –
knee contusion 10 days earlier
(22-year-old male)**

Sagittal T1: Thickening of PCL
throughout its course, discontinuity
of middle portion – inadequate
residual continuity of fibers/
synovial sheath

Fig. 4.12 a, b. PCL tear, grade III – knee contusion 2 months earlier (60-year-old male)

a, b Coronal T1: Abnormally increased signal intensity and massive thickening of circular PCL at the lateral margin of the medial condyle – cf. normal appearance in Fig. 4.1

Fig. 4.13 a, b. Midsubstance PCL tear, grade III – knee distortion 4 weeks earlier (18-year-old male)

a Sagittal T1; **b** sagittal T2*: Massive thickening and abnormal signal increase of the PCL through-out its course with central third showing extensive discontinuity including the synovial sheath on the anterior side, most clearly appreciated on relative T2-weight-ing (*arrow*)

a

b

Fig. 4.14. PCL tear, grade III, 4 months earlier (32-year-old male)

Sagittal T1: Irregular, cloudy struc-tures replacing the PCL – no fiber continuity discernible

Fig. 4.15 a, b. Old PCL tear, sustained 5 years earlier – old grade III lesion (42-year-old male)

a Sagittal T1: Nonvisualization of PCL – some residual connective tissue fibers

b Coronal T1: Round ligament structure at lateral margin of medial condyle replaced by irregular remnant – cf. normal appearance in Fig. 4.1

a

b

Fig. 4.16. Bony PCL avulsion 5 weeks earlier, intraligamentous hemorrhage (27-year-old male)

Sagittal T1: Linear signal decreases in the tibial plateau with disruption of cortical bone at the base of the PCL insertion. Contour broadening and increased signal intensity of the distal portion of the slightly compressed PCL (*arrow*)

**Fig. 4.17. Bony PCL avulsion
3 months earlier
(47-year-old female)**

Sagittal; *left* T1, *right* T2*: Avulsion
of a small triangular bone fragment
from the posteromedial tibial
plateau in the area of the base of
the PCL insertion. Fracture cleft
showing decreased signal intensity
on T1-weighted image and pronounced signal increase on relative
T2-weighting (*arrows*). Slightly
increased signal intensity and
slight contour broadening of the
distal PCL

**Fig. 4.18. Bony PCL avulsion
1 week earlier (49-year-old male)**

Sagittal; *left* T1, *right* T2*: Disruption of cortical bone in the area of
the base of the tibial PCL insertion
with mild signal decrease on
T1-weighted image and increased
signal intensity on relative
T2-weighting (*arrows*). Increased
signal intensity mainly of proximal
third of PCL on relative T2-weight-
ing. Joint effusion

Fig. 4.19 a–c. Bony PCL avulsion with slight displacement 1 week earlier, hemorrhage into adjacent soft tissue and cruciate ligament. Slight joint effusion (49-year-old male)

a Sagittal; *left* T1, *right* T2*: Avulsion of a bone fragment from the tibial PCL insertion site with slight proximal displacement by 0.5 cm. Relatively T2-weighted image shows increased signal intensity of the fracture cleft as well as of the PCL, especially of its distal half, and of the retrotibial muscle. Slight joint effusion

b Coronal T1: Avulsed bone fragment delineated against the lower-signal-intensity, curved fracture cleft (*arrow*)

c Axial T2*: Avulsed tibial bone fragment clearly identified posteriorly against the hyperintense background of the fracture cleft (*arrow*)

a

b

5 Anterior (and Posterior) Cruciate Ligament Reconstruction

5.1 Technique and Method

The imaging technique and patient positioning in evaluating graft integrity are essentially the same as for assessing the natural anterior and posterior cruciate ligaments. Supplementary thin-slice images in parasagittal or paracoronal orientations along the requisite course of the ligament should be acquired as needed.

5.2 Anatomy

Reconstruction of the cruciate ligaments is usually performed using tissue from other sites of the body as autografts. Because of numerous disadvantages, allografts and prosthetic ligaments have mostly been abandoned.

The most common graft sources in autograft reconstruction of the ACL are the patellar tendon and the hamstring tendons (semitendinosus and gracilis). In more recent approaches using the hamstring tendons, the graft is run in up to four parallel strands in order to match or even surpass the strength of the natural ligament.

The main factors determining the permanent stability of cruciate ligament substitutes are the selection of proper attachment sites that take into account the anatomic ligament attachment sites (as described in Chaps. 3 and 4 on cruciate ligaments), the anchoring of the graft near the attachment site, and the prevention of hollow space formation along the length of fixation.

Regarding graft fixation, a basic distinction is made between fixation near the insertion site and fixation distant from it. Near fixation is mainly done using foreign materials such as inference screws made of titanium or bioabsorbable polymers. It can also be done without introduction of such materials using the press-fit technique. Distant fixation is secured by anchoring screws, staples, or round/oval metal buttons.

Distant fixation has the disadvantage of requiring fixation along an extended stretch of the graft, which reduces its stiffness. There is an increasing tendency to attempt to refill hollow spaces in the bone tunnel with spongiosa, most of which is collected during drilling.

Ligament grafts are rotated on their longitudinal axis in such a way that the fibers run nearly parallel in extension and twist around each other to various extents with flexion. Deliberately overrotated grafts have not proven effective.

Ligament reconstruction is frequently combined with enlargement of the intercondylar space, in particular of the anterior roof portion, by a so-called notch plasty to ensure undiverted sliding of the graft, especially in near extension.

5.3 Normal MRI Appearance

The MRI appearance of a successfully reconstructed ACL varies with the surgical technique employed and the material used (autograft or allograft). Patellar tendon grafts are the internationally preferred material for ligament reconstruction because they are superior to prosthetic materials.

The patellar tendon graft is fixed in a tibial and femoral bone tunnel. Metallic implants or metal debris in this area often produce artifacts on MR images. In a normal graft, the bone tunnel walls are smooth and decrease in signal intensity over time. The marrow space outside the bone tunnel area shows no changes.

Postoperatively the ligament graft has absent or very low signal intensity on T1- and T2-weighted images. The formation of granulation tissue and increasing vascularization produce increasing signal intensity 6–8 months after surgery, which may mimic contour thinning. Thereafter, the graft typically returns to its earlier thickness and the signal intensity decreases again (Figs. 4.1 – 4.5).

5.4 Pathomechanism

The selection of inadequate fixation sites, long-stretched and loose fixation, large hollow spaces, and weakness of the graft material may result in secondary failure of the reconstructed cruciate ligament.

"Genuine" graft failure, however, is caused by spontaneous lengthening of the grafted tissue. Recurrent damage requires careful analysis in terms of severity in order to differentiate true repeat rupture caused by trauma from instabilities due to gradual graft failure.

Besides graft failure, scar formation limiting the range of motion is a frequent cause of postoperative complaints. Excessive fibrous tissue formation (arthrofibrosis) may be localized (local causes) or generalized (primarily autoimmune causes).

A known cause of extension loss of the knee after ACL reconstruction that results from a true mechanical block is localized anterior fibrosis. This so-called cyclops lesion is a polyp-like structure consisting of fibrous granulation tissue about 1 cm in thickness that extends anterior to and along the graft between the graft and the intercondylar wall.

5.5 Pathophysiology

The most common mistake made in ACL reconstruction is incorrect femoral fixation in the anterior portion of the lateral intercondylar wall instead of the posterior portion, typically resulting in limited knee flexion due to the increasing tension that develops with flexion.

5.6 MRI Signs of Abnormal Findings

- Assessment of the bone tunnel (femoral insertion should ideally be as posterior as possible and somewhat higher than that of the natural ligament, tibial insertion at least 2 cm anterior to the anterior margin of the PCL attachment but not in front of the projection of Blumensaat's line in knee extension – notch impingement).
- Margins of bone tunnel (blurring, lytic zones with widening of tunnel exit and entrance in about 25% of patients operated on).
- Signal intensity of tunnel (reduced signal on T1-weighting and increased signal on relative T2-weighting for up to 1 year – edema phase; increasing hypointensity of the tunnel thereafter).
- Increased signal intensity in the course of the ligament graft (focal or generalized; Fig. 5.7).
- Irregular internal structures (spreading of fibers, blurring, partial discontinuity).
- Changes in diameter (focal or generalized thickening/thinning; Fig. 5.6).
- Changes in contour (irregular, partial/complete disruption; Figs. 5.8 and 5.9).
- Changes in course (curving, kinking, abnormal orientation, retraction).
- Paraligamentous changes: hemorrhage, pseudo-mass, osteophytic processes at the roof of the intercondylar fossa or at the tibia with graft impingement.
- Rupture of graft with residual tibial ligament portion bending anteriorly toward Hoffa's fat pad while femoral ligament residues may fuse with PCL.
- Formation of fibrous granulation tissue in front of and along the ACL graft (cyclops lesion).
- Femorotibial malalignment.

5.7 MRI Grading

As of yet there is no generally accepted international classification of injuries to reconstructed cruciate ligaments.

The classification proposed by Yamato and Yamagishu (1992) distinguishes 4 categories:

Category 1: Graft not disrupted and of low signal intensity throughout its intra-articular course.

Category 2: Low signal intensity restricted to femoral graft portion.

Category 3: Low signal intensity restricted to tibial graft portion.

Category 4: Nonvisualization of low-signal-intensity structure.

5.8 Clinical Role of MRI Findings

The most important feature to be assessed is whether the graft has aligned itself with the course of the natural cruciate ligament it replaces.

Assessment has to take into account the anatomic insertion sites and the slope of the intercondylar roof, which should not impinge the graft. Ligamentous laxity of the knee with a steep Blumensaat's line may be associated with normal diversion of both the natural cruciate ligaments and ligament grafts.

A hypointense cruciate ligament graft not deviating from the anatomic course normally indicates stability of the knee. More or less hyperintense grafts, especially after over a year of healing, may suggest graft failure. But this is not necessarily the case since not all grafts showing hyperintensity at MRI are associated with knee instability.

Further Reading

Bernard M, Hertel P, Hornung H, Cierpinski T (1997) Femoral insertion of the ACL-radiographic quadrant method. Am J Knee Surg 10: 14–22

Bradley DM, Bergman AG, Dillingham MF (2000) MR imaging of cyclops lesions. AJR Am J Roentgenol 174 (3): 719–726

Cassa Pullicino VN, McCall IW, Strover AE (1994) MRI of the knee following prosthetic anterior cruciate ligament reconstruction. Clin Radiol 49 (2): 89–99

Chan KK, Resnick D, Goodwin D, Seeger LL (1999) Posteromedial tibial plateau injury including avulsion fracture of the semimembranous tendon insertion site: ancillary sign of anterior cruciate ligament tear at MR imaging. Radiology 211 (3): 754–758

Echigo J, Yoshioka H, Takahashi H, Niitsu M, Fukubayashi T, Itai Y (1999) Signal intensity changes in anterior cruciate ligament autografts: reaction to magnetic field orientation. Acad Radiol 6 (4): 206–210

Hertel P, Bernard M (1994) Vordere Kreuzbandersatzplastik – Vorteile einer metallfreien offenen Press-Fit-Operationstechnik (Einschnitttechnik) gegenüber einer arthroskopischen Unitunnel-Technik. In: Kohn D, Wirth CJ (eds) Arthroskopische versus offene Operationen. Enke, Stuttgart

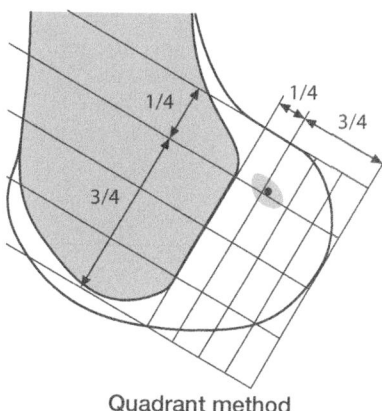

Quadrant method

Diagram 1. a Normal course of ACL; average center of tibial insertion at 43% of longitudinal tibial diameter. Modified according to Stäubli and Rauschning (1994)

Diagram 1. b Normal center of femoral insertion of ACL in the lower corner of the uppermost quadrant on strictly lateral radiographs. Quadrant method according to Bernard et al. (1997)

Hogerle S, Letsch R, Sievers KW (1998) ACL reconstruction by patellar tendon. A comparison of length by magnetic resonance imaging. Arch Orthop Trauma Surg 117 (1–2): 58–61

Horton LK, Jacobson JA, Lin-J, Hayes CW (2000) MR imaging of anterior cruciate ligament reconstruction graft. AJR Am J Roentgenol 175 (4): 1091–1097

Jansson KA, Harilainen A, Sandelin J, Karjalainen PT, Aronen HJ, Tallroth K (1999) Bone tunnel enlargement after anterior cruciate ligament reconstruction with the hamstring autograft and endobutton fixation technique. A clinical, radiographic and magnetic resonance imaging study with 2 years follow-up. Knee Surg Sports Traumatol Arthrosc 7 (5): 290–295

Joergensen U, Thomsen HS (2000) Behavior of the graft within the bone tunnels following anterior cruciate ligament reconstruction, studied by cinematic magnetic resonance imaging. Knee Surg Sports Traumatol Arthrosc 8 (1): 32–35

Kuehne JH, Durr HR, Steinborn M, Jansson V, Refior HJ (1998) Magnetic resonance imaging and knee stability following ACL reconstruction. Orthopedics 21 (1): 39–43

Lajtai G, Noszian I, Humer K, Unger F, Aitzetmuller G, Orthner E (1999) Serial magnetic resonance imaging evaluation of operative site after fixation of patellar tendon graft with bioabsorbable interference screws in anterior cruciate ligament reconstruction. Arthroscopy 15 (7): 709–718

Mariani PP, Adriani E, Bellelli A, Maresca G (1999) Magnetic resonance imaging of tunnel placement in posterior cruciate ligament reconstruction. Arthroscopy 15 (7): 733–740

Maurer EJ, Kaplan PA, Dussault RG et al. (1997) Acutely injured knee: effect of MR imaging on diagnostic and therapeutic decisions. Radiology 204 (3): 799–805

Murakami Y, Sumen Y, Ochi M, Fujimoto E, Adachi N, Ikuta Y (1998) MR evaluation of human anterior cruciate ligament autograft on oblique axial imaging. J Comput Assist Tomogr 22 (2): 270–275

Murakami Y, Sumen Y, Ochi M, Fujimoto E, Deie M, Ikuta Y (1999) Appearance of anterior cruciate ligament autografts in their tibial bone tunnels on oblique axial MRI. Magn Reson Imaging 17 (5): 679–687

Pomeranz SJ (1991) Orthopaedic MRI. JB Lippincott, Philadephia, S 68

Recht MP, Parker RD, Irizarry JM (2000) Second time around: evaluating the postoperative anterior cruciate ligament. Magn Reson Imaging Clin N Am 8 (2): 285–297

Recht MP, Piraino DW, Cohen MA, Parker RD, Bergfeld JA (1995) Localized anterior arthrofibrosis (cyclops lesion) after reconstruction of the anterior cruciate ligament: MR imaging findings. AJR Am J Roentgenol 165 (2): 383–385

Stäubli HU, Rauschning W (1994) Tibial attachment area of the anterior cruciate ligament in the extended knee position. Knee Surg Sports Traumatol Arthrosc 2: 138–146

Stoeckle U, Hoffmann R, Schwedke J, Lubrich J, Vogl T, Suedkamp NP, Haas N (1998) Anterior cruciate ligament reconstruction: the diagnostic value of MRI. Int Orthop 22 (5): 288–292

Stoeckle U, Hoffmann R, Schwedtke J, Lubrich J, Vogl T, Suedkamp NP (1997) Wertigkeit der MRT in der Beurteilung des Kreuzbandersatzes. Unfallchirurg 100 (3): 212–218

Träger JS et al. (1995) Kernspintomographie zur Beurteilung der Transplantatqualität bei Kreuzbandersatz. Sportorthopädie Sporttraumatologie 11 (4): 241–246

Uhl M, Schmidt C, Riedl S, Brado M, Kauffmann GW, Friedl W (1996) Die postoperative MRT-Morphologie des vorderen Kreuzbandes nach primärer Bandnaht oder Bandplastik. Eine prospektive Studie an 50 Patienten. Aktuelle Radiol 6 (1): 13–18

Yamato M, Yamagishi T (1992) MRI of patellar tendon anterior cruciate ligament autografts. J Comput Assist Tomogr 16 (4): 604–607

Table 5.1. Characteristic signal intensities

	T1w	T2w	T2*w	rho-w	FAT-SAT
Ligament graft postoperatively	0	0	0 – ↑	0	0
Ligament graft after 6–8 months	↑	↑↑	↑ – ↑↑	↑	↑
Ligament graft after 8 months	0	0	0	0	0
Bone tunnels up to 1 year	↑	↑ – ↑↑	↑ – ↑↑	↑	↑ – ↑↑
Bone tunnels after 1 year	0	0	0	0	0

0 No signal; ↑ low SI; ↑↑ intermediate SI; ↑↑↑ high SI.

Fig. 5.1. Intact ACL graft – reconstruction 5 months earlier (27-year-old male)

Sagittal T1: ACL graft clearly delineated as a hypointense band with smooth contours. Tibial bone tunnel likewise smoothly marginated. Isolated artifacts produced by abraded metal at the tunnel margin. Steep course of graft due to relatively posterior tibial tunnel

Fig. 5.2. Intact ACL graft – reconstruction 9 months earlier (45-year-old male)

Coronal T1: ACL graft depicted as a hypointense band with smooth margins in the center of the joint. Steep intercondylar roof, femoral insertion at 60% of length of roof (*not shown*)

Fig. 5.3. Intact ACL graft, minimal edema – reconstruction $^1/_2$ year earlier (31-year-old female)

Sagittal; *left* T1, *right* T2*: Normal course of graft with isolated intraligamentous linear hyperintensities. Slight joint effusion. Course parallel to intercondylar roof (Blumensaat's line)

Fig. 5.4. Intact ACL graft – reconstruction ¹/₂ year earlier (31-year-old male)

Sagittal T1: Graft thinner along its intra-articular course (*arrow*) but with intact continuity. Isolated artifacts caused by metal debris at posterior margin of tibial tunnel and distally by osteosynthesis material. Triangular area of increased signal on T1-weighting indicates irritation of proximal patellar tendon bed following harvesting of graft

Fig. 5.5 a, b. ACL reconstruction using telos graft 2 months earlier (30-year-old male)

a Sagittal T1; b parasagittal T1 along the course of the tibial tunnel: Telos graft depicted as a delicate track-like structure in the joint space and tibial tunnel. Intact patellar tendon. Midsubstance tears of Hoffa's fat pad with linear to broader areas of increased signal intensity. Proper course of reconstructed cruciate ligament (over-the-top route)

a

b

Fig. 5.6. Pronounced atrophy of ACL graft – reconstruction 1 year earlier (35-year-old male)

Sagittal T1: Only faint depiction of tibial half of ACL graft proximal to the bone tunnel (*arrow*), continuity intact. Notch impingement resulting from placement of tibial tunnel too far anteriorly (Blumensaat's line)

Fig. 5.7 a, b. Partial tear of ACL graft with considerable edema formation; reconstruction 8 months earlier – clinically stable (24-year-old female)

a Sagittal T1; **b** sagittal T2*: Considerable thickening of intra-articular portions of ACL graft with poorly discernible fibers – doubtful continuity on MRI – no surgery

a

b

Fig. 5.8. Tear of ACL graft 4 weeks earlier – reconstruction 2 $\frac{1}{2}$ years earlier (32-year-old male)

Sagittal; *left* T1, *right* T2*: Highly irregular/discontinuous intra-articular fibers of ACL graft – most conspicuous on relative T2-weighting (*right image*). Unequivocal morphology (no repeat surgery)

Fig. 5.9. Tear of ACL graft on the day before (23-year-old male)

Sagittal; *left* and *right* T1: No continuity of intra-articular course of ACL graft

Fig. 5.10 a – c see p. 65

Fig. 5.11. Intact ACL and PCL grafts – reconstruction 2 years earlier (24-year-old female)

Sagittal T1: Depiction of hypointense structures of reconstructed ACL (*arrow*) and PCL (*arrowhead*) within the joint space. Tibial insertion of PCL graft positioned somewhat too far anteriorly

Fig. 5.10 a – c. Proximal atrophy of PCL graft – reconstruction 2 years earlier (36-year-old female)

a, b Sagittal T1; **c** sagittal T2*: Low signal intensity of PCL graft over extended stretch including portion inside tunnel. Poor visualization only of proximal part immediately distal to femoral tunnel entrance on T1-weighting (*arrows*). Relatively T2-weighted image shows delicate residual continuity of this area at anterior margin anterior to an adjacent metal artifact (*arrow* in **c**)

a

b

c

d

Fig. 5.12 a–d. Highly atrophied, lax PCL graft following recurrent tear with instability; insufficient residual continuity – reconstruction 4 months earlier (22-year-old male)

a, b Sagittal T1: Intra-articular course of PCL graft no longer clearly discernible. Likewise only abnormal high-signal-intensity residual thin structures within the tibial tunnel (*arrow*)

c, d Sagittal T2*: Course of graft again only just barely visualized with very hyperintense signal – isolated fiber portions can be identified (*arrows*). Slight edema of anterior parts of Hoffa's fat pad with increased signal intensity on relative T2-weighting

6 Medial and Lateral Collateral Ligaments

6.1 Technique and Method

The medial and lateral collateral ligaments can best be imaged using T1- and T2-weighted sequences in coronal and axial orientations.

6.2 Anatomy

The medial collateral ligament (MCL) is a flat band that passes from the medial femoral epicondyle to the medial tibial metaphysis below the pes anserinus. It is about 12 cm in length, running 4 cm above and 8 cm below the joint cleft.

Anatomically, the MCL consists of a superficial layer that serves as a stabilizer and a deep layer that contributes to the anchoring of the menisci. The posterior portions of both layers blend into each other to form the posterior oblique ligament, which extends from the femoral epicondyle to the attachment of the semimembranosus tendon.

The lateral collateral ligament (LCL) is a cord of pencil thickness that arises from the lateral femoral epicondyle and passes in a slightly posterior direction to insert into the tip of the fibula. It is straight in extension and crossed inferiorly by the popliteus tendon, which, with the knee extended, inserts into the lateral femoral condyle slightly anteriorly and distally to the LCL.

Another part of the lateral ligament structure is the arcuate ligament, which arises anteromedially to the fibular insertion of the LCL and arches across the popliteus tendon as it proceeds to the lateral femoral condyle. Between the arcuate ligament and the LCL pass the lateral inferior geniculate vessels.

6.3 Normal MRI Appearance

The MCL and the structurally much more complex LCL are depicted as homogeneous structures of low or absent signal intensity. Their femoral and tibial insertion sites cannot be differentiated from intact cortical bone.

A slender bursa of higher signal intensity is embedded between the MCL and the medial meniscus. The two collateral ligaments have a fan-like structure (Figs. 6.1, 6.7, 6.13, and 6.16).

6.4 Pathomechanism

MCL injuries are caused by abduction and/or external rotation mechanisms and may present as femoral or tibial avulsions or areas of fiber spreading.

The deep layer of the MCL can avulse from its capsular attachment or the base of the meniscus independently of the superficial layer. Multilevel injuries may occur. Posterior extension of a rupture results in concomitant damage of the posterior oblique ligament or even of the entire posterior capsule.

Avulsion of the LCL from its femoral or fibular insertion is frequently associated with concomitant injury to the popliteus tendon and the arcuate ligament.

Avulsions from the anterolateral capsule not involving the LCL are frequently associated with the presence of a small bony fragment (Segond fragment), suggesting concomitant rupture of the ACL.

6.5 Pathophysiology

Both collateral ligaments serve to restrain varus-valgus stress and/or rotation forces in the lateral compartment of the knee. Collateral injuries are typically treated conservatively. Only in patients with complex injuries does it make sense to stabilize collateral ligament tears as well.

6.6 MRI Signs of Abnormal Findings

- Increased signal intensity on T1- and T2-weighting (focal or generalized).
- Internal structural irregularities (spreading and undulation of fibers, blurring, partial disruption).
- Changes in diameter (focal or generalized thickening/thinning).
- Changes in external contour (irregular, partial/complete contour disruption).
- Paraligamentous changes: fluid collection in adjacent subcutaneous tissue, possibly extending to the popliteal muscle, and indicated by increased signal intensity on relatively T2-weighted images and reduced signal intensity on T1-weighting.

6.7 MRI Grading of Collateral Ligament Injuries

Based on the widely accepted international classification of ligament injuries of the American Medical Association, the following grades of collateral ligament injuries are distinguished on MRI:

I. Strain/Subtle Midsubstance Tear

Only intraligamentous structural changes. Increased signal intensity on T1- and T2*-weighted images, bulk of fibers intact, and unimpaired external configuration (unchanged contour, thickness, length; Figs. 6.2, 6.3, and 6.8).

II. Partial Tear

Increased signal intensity in both sequences and thickening with onion-like appearance (intraligamentous edema/hemorrhage), contour and fiber irregularities or partial discontinuity. MCL may show some separation from meniscus (Figs. 6.4–6.6, 6.9–6.11, 6.14, 6.15, and 6.17).

III. Complete Tear

Considerable increases in signal intensity, discontinuity, potential retraction. MCL may show more extensive separation from meniscus. Large fluid collections in surrounding structures, possibly including perimuscular/intramuscular area (Figs. 6.12 and 6.18).

Chronic Injury

Chronic collateral injuries present with a reduced signal intensity and smoothed contour distention. Areas of hyperintensity may indicate intraligamentous fat accumulation. MRI is inferior to radiography in identifying intraligamentous or capsular calcifications (signal voids or curved areas of increased signal intensity through inclusion of ferromagnetic substances) (see Fig. 6.18).

Table 6.1. Characteristic signal intensities

	T1w	T2w	T2*w	rho-w	FAT-SAT
Collateral ligaments	0	0	0 – ↑	0	0
Strain	↑	↑ – ↑↑	↑	↑	↑
Tear	↑	↑↑ – ↑↑↑	↑↑ – ↑↑↑	↑↑	↑↑ – ↑↑↑

0 No signal; ↑ low SI; ↑↑ intermediate SI; ↑↑↑ high SI.

6.8 Clinical Role of MRI Findings

MRI has a crucial role in determining the localization of MCL and LCL tears but depends on the guidance of clinical findings, particularly the site of pain on palpation.

Moreover, MRI can provide useful evidence confirming defined attachment ruptures, help in determining the level of surgical access, and contribute prognostic information on the outcome of reattachment.

Further Reading

Farooki S, Seeger LL (1999) Magnetic resonance imaging in the evaluation of ligament injuries. Skeletal Radiol 28 (2): 61–74

Irizarry JM, Recht MP (1997) MR imaging of the knee ligaments and the postoperative knee. Radiol Clin North Am 35 (1): 45–76

Marks PH, Chew BH (1995) Magnetic resonance imaging of knee ligaments. Am J Knee Surg 8 (4): 181–187

Mirowitz SA, Shu HH (1994) MR imaging evaluation of knee collateral ligaments and related injuries: comparison of T1-weighted, T2-weighted, and fat-saturated T2-weighted sequences – correlation with clinical findings. J Magn Reson Imaging 4 (5): 725–732

Niitsu M, Ikeda K, Iijima T, Ochiai N, Noguchi M, Itai Y (1999) MR imaging of Pellegrini-Stieda disease. Radiat Med 17 (6): 405–409

Patel JJ (1999) Intra-articular entrapment of the medial collateral ligament: radiographic and MRI findings. Skeletal Radiol 28 (11): 658–660

Patten RM, Richardson ML, Zink Brody G, Rolfe BA (1994) The semimembranosus-tibial collateral ligament bursa. Anatomical study and magnetic resonance imaging. J Bone Joint Surg Am 76 (9): 1322–1327

Pomeranz SJ (1991) Orthopaedic MRI. JB Lippincott, Philadelphia, pp 73–75

Pope TL Jr (1996) MR imaging of knee ligaments. J South Orthop Assoc 5 (1): 46–62

Rasenberg EI, Lemmens JA, von Kampen A, Schoots F, Bloo HJ, Wagemakers HP, Blankevoort L (1995) Grading medial collateral ligament injury: comparison of MR imaging and instrumented valgus-varus laxity test-device. A prospective double-blind patient study. Eur J Radiol 21 (1): 18–24

Rubin DA, Kettering JM, Towers JD, Britton CA (1998) MR imaging of knees having isolated and combined ligament injuries. AJR Am J Roentgenol 170 (5): 1207–1213

Yao L, Dungan D, Seeger LL (1994) MR imaging of tibial collateral ligament injury: comparison with clinical examination. Skeletal Radiol 23 (7): 521–524

**Fig. 6.1. Normal MCL, right knee
(19-year-old female)**

Coronal T1: MCL depicted as a
delicate low-signal-intensity structure with smooth margins in the
vicinity of the medial condyle
(*arrow*). Sliding fat/intraligamen-
tous fat lamella between the
superficial and deep layers of the
ligament (*arrowhead*)

**Fig. 6.2a, b. Partial MCL tear,
right knee, grade I – distortion
3 days earlier (59-year-old male)**

a Coronal T1: MCL showing thickening, increased signal intensity,
and partial discontinuity at femoral
insertion

b Axial T2*: Fibers of MCL
markedly hyperintense and partly
discontinuous. Slightly increased
signal intensity of adjoining
anteromedial subcutaneous structures

a

b

Fig. 6.3 a, b. Partial MCL tear, right knee, grade I (41-year-old male)

a Coronal T1: MCL showing slight (to moderate) thickening and partial fiber discontinuity

b Coronal T2*: Pronounced signal increase of the edematous and partly discontinuous MCL (*arrow*)

a

b

Fig. 6.4. Partial MCL tear, right knee, grade II – lateral knee contusion 3 months earlier (26-year-old male)

Coronal T1: MCL with pronounced thickening of femoral portion and circumscribed fiber discontinuity (*arrow*)

a

b

Fig. 6.5 a, b. Nearly complete MCL tear at tibial insertion, right knee, grade II–III – distortion 4 days earlier (35-year-old male)

a, b Coronal T1: MCL abnormally increased in signal intensity and nearly completely elevated from its tibial insertion. Considerable fiber discontinuity close to complete rupture. Partial thickening of femoral MCL portion (*arrow* in **b**)

Fig. 6.6. Older MCL tear at tibial insertion, right knee, grade III, 3 months earlier (23-year-old male)

Coronal T1: Tibial insertion of MCL no longer clearly discernible due to thickening in this area; similar appearance on subsequent sections (*not shown*)

Fig. 6.7. Normal appearance of MCL, left knee (34-year-old male)

Coronal T1: Black band with smooth, delicate margins at medial condyle (*arrow*)

Fig. 6.8. Partial MCL tear, left knee, grade I – II, 3 weeks earlier (35-year-old male)

Coronal T1: MCL shows marked thickening, increased signal intensity, and partial discontinuity at medial condyle

ⓐ

ⓑ

Fig. 6.9 a, b. (Subtotal) MCL tear at femoral insertion, left knee, grade II – III; discreet partial LCL tear, grade I – distortion 3 months earlier (45-year-old male)

a Coronal T1; b coronal T2*: Considerable signal increase and fiber discontinuities of proximal MCL – most conspicuous on relatively T2-weighted image. Anterior and posterior portions intact (*not shown*). Fluid exudation into subcutaneous fatty tissue in the area of most pronounced MCL damage. LCL showing mild corresponding changes. Minute peripheral tear of medial meniscus without distinct meniscoligamentous separation

Fig. 6.10. Extensive partial MCL tear, left knee, grade II – distortion 10 days earlier (17-year-old male)

Coronal T1: Considerable fiber discontinuity of central portion of MCL with intact outer fascia. Small peripheral partial tear of medial meniscus (*arrow*)

Fig. 6.11 a, b. Subtotal MCL tear, left knee, grade II – III; menisco-ligamentous separation with delicate peripheral partial tear of medial meniscus. Strain/subtle partial tear of LCL, grade I – discreet tear of base of lateral meniscus (51-year-old male)

a, b Sagittal T2*: Distention, thickening, and increased signal intensity of MCL with pronounced partial discontinuity, most conspicuous in **b** (*arrow*). Tiny triangular contour defect in periphery of medial meniscus and increased distance from collateral ligament (**a**). Slight reactive edema of lateral soft tissue near iliotibial tract with increased signal intensity on relative T2-weighting (LCL injury not shown). Discreet contour disruption of inferior surface of abnormally broad anterior horn of lateral meniscus

a

b

Fig. 6.12 a – c. MCL tear, left knee, grade III; contusion of lateral condyle (16-year-old male)

a, b Coronal T1: Massive broadening of MCL with nearly complete discontinuity, especially in central (**b**) and distal (**a**) portions. Reduced signal intensity of lateral aspect of lateral condyle on T1-weighted image consistent with circumscribed microfracture zone without disruption of cortical bone

c Axial T2*: Very pronounced signal increase and fiber discontinuity of MCL and increased signal intensity of adjoining anteromedial subcutaneous structures due to edema

a

b

c

Fig. 6.13. Normal LCL, right knee, small tear of posterior horn of medial meniscus (31-year-old male)

Coronal T1: LCL depicted as a delicate, hypointense structure between the lateral condyle and the head of fibula (*arrow*)

Fig. 6.14a, b. Partial LCL tear, right knee, grade I – II (29-year-old male)

a, b Coronal T1: Markedly thickened and tortuous LCL with higher signal intensity than other ligamentous structures (*arrows*)

a

b

a

b

c

d

Fig. 6.15 a – d. Chronic partial LCL tear, right knee, grade I – II – distortion 1 year earlier; emerging secondary ganglion cyst (57-year-old male)

a, b Coronal T1: Thickening and distention of LCL fibers with partial distal discontinuity. Ganglion-like fluid accumulations with slightly convex configuration at laterobasal margin (*arrow*). Increased-signal-intensity edema of popliteus tendon attachment on T1-weighting (**b**)

c Coronal T2*; **d** axial T2*: Both images showing markedly increased signal intensity of the thickened LCL portion and of the popliteus tendon attachment (**c**)

**Fig. 6.16a, b. Normal appearance
of LCL, left knee
(33-year-old female)**

a, b Coronal T1: Rather slender LCL
with otherwise normal hypointensity and smooth margins
throughout its course

a

b

Fig. 6.17 a, b. Partial LCL tear, left knee, grade I – II – distortion 2 weeks earlier (40-year-old male)

a, b Coronal T1: Moderately increased signal intensity of LCL with spreading of fibers and thickening

Fig. 6.18 a, b. Subtotal tears of LCL and PCL, left knee, grade II – III; discreet partial tears of ACL and MCL, grade I – distortion 3 weeks earlier (29-year-old male)

a, b Coronal T1: Massive thickening with nearly complete discontinuity of proximal and distal portions of LCL including the popliteal tendon. Markedly increased signal intensity of these areas (*arrows*). Considerably increased transverse diameter of PCL at lateral margin of medial condyle (*arrowheads*) – cf. normal appearance in Fig. 6.1. Only slight irregularities of ACL and MCL at femoral insertions (**a**)

7 Complex Knee Injuries, Fractures, Patellar Dislocation

7.1 Technique and Method

Next to T1-weighted imaging, fat-suppressed sequences are most useful. Additional imaging with intravenous contrast medium administration may be helpful in identifying detached or displaced fragments. However, most cases do not require contrast-enhanced imaging and the examiner must be aware that the contrast medium may in fact obscure bone marrow edema.

7.2 Anatomy

All structures of the knee may be affected. Bony, cartilaginous, capsular, and ligamentous injuries may occur.

7.3 Normal MRI Appearance

The normal subchondral marrow space is of intermediate signal intensity on T2-weighted images, hyperintense on T1-weighting, and almost black on fat-suppressed sequences.

7.4 Pathomechanism

In assessing complex knee injuries, it is important to obtain a history of the mechanisms of injury. If need be, the patient should demonstrate how the injury occurred. This will often reveal a common cause that easily explains concomitant ligament and bone injuries.

7.5 Pathophysiology

A straight valgus opening mechanism may cause simultaneous or successive rupture of the medial collateral ligament and a compression fracture or simple bone bruise of the lateral joint (mainly of the tibial plateau).

Patellar dislocation is characterized by cartilage and bone injuries of the medial patellar margin and the lateral femoral condyle with concomitant local hemorrhage in the area of the medial retinaculum between the medial femoral condyle and the medial patellar margin. Splintered osteochondral fragments may be present in the joint space.

7.6 MRI Signs of Abnormal Findings

Discreet Bone Contusions (Bone Bruises)

Bone bruises are associated with circumscribed intraosseous edema which appears on MRI as a mild diffuse signal decrease on T1-weighted images and increased signal intensity on relatively T2-weighted or fat-suppressed sequences.

The signal abnormalities associated with discreet changes recede on spin-echo images within 2–4 weeks but persist much longer on fat-suppressed T2-weighted images (asymptomatic). Depending on the severity of the injury and the study reported, signal abnormalities last for 3 to 10 months.

A crucial aspect is the assessment of cortical disruptions and chondral involvement, since there is some tendency for patients with concomitant osteochondral damage to develop osteochondritis dissecans (Figs. 7.1, 7.3, 7.7, and 7.17).

Genuine Fractures

Genuine fractures are depicted as linear signal decreases with cortical bone disruption and possibly with displacement. There is rapid development of hemarthrosis, identified on T1-weighted images by a slightly higher signal than serous fluid. T2-weighted images cannot distinguish blood from serous effusion (Figs. 7.2, 7.7, 7.9, 7.11 – 7.16).

Chronic Fractures

The majority of chronic fractures are characterized in all sequences by hypointense, inhomogeneous lesions representing sclerosis of the medullary space and fibrous tissue (Fig. 7.21).

Fatigue Fractures

Fatigue or stress fractures are a specific type of fracture combining acute and chronic components, depicted on MRI as hypointense and hyperintense signal changes, frequently in the form of lines or bands in typical location, especially in the proximal tibia (Figs. 7.18 – 7.20).

Pathologic Fractures

Pathologic fractures caused by tumor or metastatic growth require contrast-enhanced imaging only in cases where an improved assessment of extensive extraosseous invasion of soft tissue is required.

Patellar Dislocation

Patellar dislocation frequently occurs in patients with predisposing factors (high-riding patella, Wiberg types III and IV, hunter's cap, and/or flattening of the articular surface of the femoral condyle in patellofemoral dysplasia). Typically associated with bone bruises of the lateral condyle (82%) and medial patellar margin (41%), chondral/osteochondral involvement (73%), and hemarthrosis (95%).

Additionally associated with abnormal signal increases and possibly discontinuities of medial retinaculum as well as bleeding into surrounding structures (Figs. 7.4 – 7.8).

Posttraumatic Osteonecrosis

Bone necrosis is characterized on T1-weighted images by extensive intraosseous signal decreases – possibly being most prominent in subchondral bone – and by increased signal intensities of the abnormal areas on relatively T2-weighted images or fat-suppressed sequences (Figs. 7.22 and 7.23).

Ligament Injuries

For the specific signs of ligament injuries see the respective chapters on patellar tendon (Chap. 1), quadriceps tendon (Chap. 2), anterior cruciate ligament (Chap. 3), posterior cruciate ligament (Chap. 4), cruciate ligament reconstruction (Chap. 5), and collateral ligaments (Chap. 6).

Table 7.1. Characteristic signal intensities

	T1w	T2w	T2*w	rho-w	FAT-SAT
Compact/ spongy bone	0	0	0	0	0
Marrow (yellow)	↑↑↑	↑ – ↑↑	0 – ↑	↑↑	0
Bone contusion	↑ – 0	↑	↑↑ – ↑↑↑	↑ – ↑↑	↑↑ – ↑↑↑

0 No signal; ↑ low SI; ↑↑ intermediate SI; ↑↑↑ high SI.

7.7 Clinical Role of MRI Findings

The significance of multiple bone bruises first detected by MRI awaits conclusive analysis as few long-term studies are available.

Faber et al. (1999) found reductions in the thickness of articular cartilage and signal changes in the area of bone bruises 6 years after anterior cruciate ligament rupture. The impact of such osteochondral contusions on primary patient care remains to be determined.

Further Reading

Arndt WF III, Truax AL, Barnett FM, Simmons GE, Brown DC (1996) MR diagnosis of bone contusions of the knee: comparison of coronal T2-weighted fast spin-echo with fat saturation and fast spin-echo STIR images with conventional STIR images. AJR Am J Roentgenol 166 (1): 119–124

Brophy DP, O'Malley M, Lui D, Denison B, Eustace S (1996) MR imaging of tibial plateau fractures. Clin Radiol 51 (12): 873–878

Faber KJ, Dill JR, Amendola A, Thain L, Spouge A, Fowler PJ (1999) Occult osteochondral lesions after anterior cruciate ligament rupture. Six-year magnetic resonance imaging follow-up study. Am J Sports Med 27 (4): 489–494

Hinshaw MH, Tuite MJ, De Smet AA (2000) "Dem bones": osteochondral injuries of the knee. Magn Reson Imaging Clin N Am 8 (2): 335–348

Johnson DL, Urban WP Jr, Caborn DN, Vanarthos WJ, Carlson CS (1998) Articular cartilage changes seen with magnetic resonance imaging-detected bone bruises associated with acute anterior cruciate ligament rupture. Am J Sports Med 26 (3): 409–414

Kaplan PA, Gehl RH, Dussault RG, Anderson MW, Diduch DR (1999) Bone contusions of the posterior lip of the medial tibial plateau (contrecoup injury) and associated internal derangements of the knee at MR imaging. Radiology 211(3):747–753

Kim CW, Jaramillo D, Hresko MT (1997) MRI demonstration of occult purely chondral fractures of the tibia: a potential mimic of meniscal tears. Pediatr Radiol 27 (9): 765–766

Kramer J, Scheurecker A, Mohr E (1995) Osteochondrale Läsionen. Radiologe 35 (2): 109–116

Kreitner KF, Grebe P, Runkel M, Schadmand Fischer S, Meurer A (1995) Stellenwert der MR-Tomographie bei traumatischen Patellaluxationen. Rofo Fortschr Geb Röntgenstr Neuen Bildgeb Verfahr 163 (1): 32–37

Mathis CE, Noonan K, Kayes K (1998) "Bone bruises" of the knee: a review. Iowa Orthop J 8: 112–117

Miller MD, Osborne JR, Gordon WT, Hinkin DT, Brinker MR (1998) the natural history of bone bruises. A prospective study of magnetic resonance imaging-detected trabecular microfractures in patients with isolated medial collateral ligament injuries. Am J Sports Med 26 (1): 15–19

Munshi M, Davidson M, MacDonald PB, Froese W, Sutherland K (2000) The efficacy of magnetic resonance imaging in acute knee injuries. Clin J Sport Med 19 (1): 34–39

Newberg AH, Witzner SM (1994) Bone bruises: their patterns and significance. Semin Ultrasound CT MR 15 (5): 396–409

Pinar H, Akseki D, Kovanlikaya I, Arac S, Bozkurt M (1997) Bone bruises detected by magnetic resonance imaging following lateral ankle sprains. Knee Surg Sports Traumatol Arthrosc 5 (2): 113–117

Ryu KN, Jaovisidha S, De Maeseneer M, Jacobson J, Sartoris DJ, Resnick D (1997) Evolving stages of lipohemarthrosis of the knee. Sequential magnetic resonance imaging findings in cadavers with clinical correlation. Invest Radiol 32 (1): 7–11

Starok M, Lenchik L, Trudell D, Resnick D (1997) Normal patellar retinaculum: MR and sonographic imaging with cadaveric correlation. AJR Am J Roentgenol 168 (6): 1493–1499

Yu JS, Cook PA (1996) Magnetic resonance imaging (MRI) of the knee: a pattern approach for evaluating bone marrow edema. Crit Rev Diagn Imaging 37 (4): 261–303

Fig. 7.1 a – c. Microfracture of anteromedial patella – anterior knee contusion 3 weeks earlier (27-year-old male)

a Sagittal T1: Mild signal decrease of anterobasal patella segments (*arrow*)

b Sagittal T2*; **c** axial T2*: Both images show pronounced signal increase of anterobasal patella segments (*arrows*) and slight signal increase of subcutaneous structures in front of patella

a

b

c

Fig. 7.2. Patellar fracture, contusion 1 week earlier (17-year-old male)

Axial T2*: Vertical contour disruption of the mediobasal patella with linear signal increase surrounded by zones of slightly less increased signal on relatively T2-weighted image

Fig. 7.3 a – d see p. 88

Fig. 7.4. Strain of medial retinaculum following patellar subluxation 3 months earlier in a patient with patellofemoral dysplasia (patella alta, Wiberg type III, and abnormal angulation – 17-year-old male)

Axial T2*: Discreet signal increase of medial retinaculum (*arrow*). Flat hunter's cap with slight residual lateral dislocation and pronounced tilting

Fig. 7.5. Partial tear of medial retinaculum following repositioning of dislocated patella 3 days earlier, hunter's cap (11-year-old boy)

Axial T2*: Medial retinaculum showing markedly increased signal intensity and slight thickening but hardly any discontinuity (*arrow*). Articular cartilage thickened on lateral facet and slightly irregular on medial facet. Slight joint effusion

a

b

c

d

Fig. 7.3 a – d. Microfracture of lateral condyle following patellar dislocation on the day before; hemarthrosis with fluid level (12-year-old girl)

a Coronal T1; c sagittal T1: Both images show mild signal decrease of anterobasal portions of medial condyle epiphysis without disruption of cortical bone. Joint fluid of higher signal intensity than purely serous fluid on T1-weighting. Vertical fluid level (*arrowheads* in c)

b Axial T2*; d sagittal T2*: Both images show increased signal intensity of anterobasal lateral condyle. Again clearly discernible fluid level within the hyperintense joint fluid (*arrowheads*). Laterally displaced and tilted hunter's cap with flattening of the femoral articular surface, a constellation encouraging dislocation. Strain of posteromedial retinaculum with contour blurring (b)

Figs. 7.4 and 7.5 see p. 87

Fig. 7.6. Extensive partial tear of medial retinaculum associated with patellar dislocation 2 weeks earlier (46-year-old male)

Axial T2*: Medial retinaculum near patella showing considerably increased signal intensity, contour thickening, and pronounced partial discontinuity. Joint effusion. No lateral dislocation or tilting of patella

Fig. 7.7. Partial tear of medial retinaculum, infraction of medial patella, and discreet bone bruise of lateral condyle following repositioning of dislocated patella 2 weeks earlier in a patient with hunter's cap (25-year-old male)

Axial T2*: Triangular contour depression of inferomedial patellar margin with surrounding signal increase on relative T2-weighting (*arrow*). Slight corresponding changes also of lateral margin of lateral condyle without cortical bone disruption (*arrowhead*). Residual lateral patellar displacement without major tilting. Pronounced thickening, increased signal intensity, and partial discontinuity of medial retinaculum. Slightly irregular articular cartilage on medial facet. Slight reactive effusion

Fig. 7.8. Tear of medial retinaculum/partial tear of anterior medial collateral ligament following patellar dislocation 5 days earlier in a patient with hunter's cap (44-year-old female)

Axial T2*: Highly irregular patellar attachment of medial retinaculum with contour disruption but without bone involvement (*arrow*). Lateral patellar subluxation. Considerable reactive effusion

a

b

c

d

Fig. 7.9 a – d. Osteochondral fracture of anterior medial condyle 4 days earlier (37-year-old male)

a Sagittal T1: Anterior surface of medial condyle showing a slightly impacted bone fragment with small step formation. Depiction of hypointense, slightly blurred fracture cleft (*arrow*)

b Sagittal T2*, **c, d** axial T2*: All three images show increased signal intensity of the bony defect zone, especially of the fracture margin. Chondral irregularities anteriorly (**c, d**). Moderate joint effusion (**b**)

Fig. 7.10a–c. Small osteolysis of lateral condyle following thorn/sting injury 3 months earlier (33-year-old male)

a Sagittal T1; **b** sagittal T2*; **c** axial T2*: Ovoid area of fluid intensity in the anterior margin of the lateral condyle with a delicate, tubular connection to the joint space (**b**). Pronounced joint effusion

a

b

c

a

b

Fig. 7.11 a, b. Fracture of distal femur just under 4 months earlier (31-year-old male)

a Coronal T1: Mostly vertically oriented line of decreased signal intensity in the distal femoral metaphyseal/epiphyseal region with extension to the joint surface (*arrow*)

b Axial T2*: Obliquely oriented line of increased signal intensity surrounded by mild sclerosis depicted as absent signal intensity and delicate disruption of cortical bone at the anterior margin of the intercondylar notch (*arrow*). Slight reactive effusion

a

b

c

d

Fig. 7.12 a–d. Extensive tibial plateau contusion with infraction; contusion of anterior margin of medial condyle; lipo-hemarthrosis – knee contusion/distortion 2 weeks earlier (15-year-old female)

a Coronal T1; **b** sagittal T1: Both images show partly diffuse decreases in signal intensity of the tibial plateau with linear signal reduction anteromedially including a small step formation below the level of the articular surface anteriorly (*arrow* in **b**). More posteriorly, the abnormal area extends to the joint surface but without cortical bone disruption or chondral involvement. Almost no signal decrease of the anterior margin of the medial condyle basally (*arrowhead* in **b**)

c Sagittal T2*: Pronounced signal increase of tibial fracture zones – again with clearly seen step formation at the anterior tibial margin (*arrow*). Slightly increased signal intensity in anterobasal aspect of medial condyle. Vertical fluid level (*arrowhead*)

d Axial T2*: Horizontal fluid level with three layers: anterior layer: fat – extremely hypointense in this sequence; central layer: serous fluid – markedly hyperintense; posterior layer: settled blood components – less markedly hyperintense

a

b

Fig. 7.13 a, b. Impression fracture of lateral tibial plateau; lateral meniscal tear – knee distortion 2 weeks earlier (45-year-old male)

a Coronal T1: Depression of anterior tibial plateau with markedly reduced signal intensity on T1-weighted image. In addition, laterobasal contour irregularities of lateral meniscus. Medial collateral ligament slightly thickened with marked edema in distal portion

b Sagittal T2*: Pronounced signal increase of anterolateral tibial plateau and delineation of a bony portion of the base of eminence (*arrowhead*). Basolateral contour defect of lateral meniscus. Joint effusion. Pronounced signal increase of medial collateral ligament with partial elevation of tibial insertion

Fig. 7.14a, b. Impression fracture of posterolateral tibial plateau – knee distortion 5 days earlier (26-year-old female)

a Sagittal T1; **b** sagittal T2*: Impacted tibial plateau fragment with basal convexity in posterolateral aspect with step formation (almost 3 mm) (*arrow* in **b**) and local disruption of articular cartilage. Fracture lines showing decreased signal intensity on T1-weighting and increased signal on relative T2-weighting. Moderate joint effusion

a

b

c

d

Fig. 7.15 a–d. Infraction/microfracture of lateral tibia and fibula; tear of anterior cruciate ligament, grade III; tear of lateral meniscal posterior horn; hemarthrosis – severe knee distortion/contusion 1 week earlier (23-year-old male)

a Coronal T1: Reduced signal intensity of lateral tibial plateau and proximal fibula around epiphyseal line. Lateral meniscal posterior horn showing vertical contour disruption (*arrow*). Anterior cruciate ligament abnormally thickened and increased in signal intensity in portion at medial margin of lateral condyle (*arrowhead*); cf. normal appearance in Figs. 4.1, 6.1, 6.7, 6.13, and 6.16

b Sagittal T1: Abnormally thickened anterior cruciate ligament with abnormal angulation of proximal, discontinuous portion. Effusion with relatively hyperintense areas due to blood components. Signal of these areas higher than that of adjacent patellar articular cartilage. Mildly inhomogeneous signal of tibial plateau without cortical involvement

c Sagittal T2*: Mild increases in signal intensity of posterolateral areas of tibia and of proximal fibula (*arrowheads*)

d Axial T2*: Distinct fluid level between settled blood components and fluid/fatty areas (*arrow*)

Fig. 7.16a, b. Infraction of fibular head; minimal contusion/infraction of posterolateral tibial plateau – indirect knee contusion 4 weeks earlier (28-year-old male)

a Coronal T1: Markedly reduced signal intensity of medial portions of fibular head with disruption of cortex and slight impression of mediobasal margin (*arrow*). Very discreet signal reduction of posterolateral tibial plateau (*arrowhead*). Lateral collateral ligament and popliteus tendon clearly delineated

b Sagittal T1: Partly diffuse, partly linear signal decrease of fibular head in the fracture area (*arrow*). Almost completely horizontal signal reduction of tibial plateau near cortex (*arrowhead*)

a

b

a

b

c

d

Fig. 7.17a–d. Tears of anterior cruciate ligament and medial collateral ligament, grade III; partial tear of lateral collateral ligament, grade II; displaced lateral meniscal tear; microfracture of posterolateral tibial plateau – knee distortion 2 weeks earlier (34-year-old male)

a Coronal T1: Abnormal thickening of femoral anterior cruciate ligament insertion at medial margin of lateral condyle (cf. normal appearance in Figs. 4.1, 6.1, 6.7, 6.13, and 6.16). Medial collateral ligament discontinuous at tibial insertion (*arrowhead*) and rarefied at femoral insertion. Fragmented lateral meniscal posterior horn (*arrow*); slightly reduced signal intensity of posterolateral tibial plateau

b Coronal T1: Discontinuous tibial insertion of medial collateral ligament (*arrowhead*; cf. normal appearance in Figs. 6.1 and 6.7); almost completely discontinuous fibular insertion of lateral collateral ligament (*arrow*; cf. normal appearance in Figs. 6.13 and 6.16)

c Sagittal T1: Lateral meniscal posterior horn just barely discernible. Slightly reduced signal intensity of posterolateral tibial plateau

d Sagittal T2*: Discontinuity of anterior cruciate ligament with abnormally increased signal intensity. Defects of Hoffa's fat pad. Joint effusion

Fig. 7.18 a, b. Tibial march fracture – 8-km hike 6 weeks earlier (43-year-old male)

a Coronal T1; b sagittal T1: Both images show broad line of reduced signal intensity nearly horizontal in orientation in the medial tibial plateau around the epiphyseal line

a

b

Fig. 7.19a, b. March/fatigue fracture of medial tibia (48-year-old male)

a Coronal T1: Rather wide, curvilinear decrease in signal intensity of the proximal medial tibia distal to the partly discernible epiphyseal line

b Sagittal T2*: Nearly horizontal, slightly irregular increase in signal intensity of the proximal medial tibia on relative T2-weighting (*arrow*)

a

b

c

d

Fig. 7.20a–d. March/fatigue fracture of medial tibia; tear of medial meniscus (69-year-old female)

a, b Coronal T1; **c** sagittal T1: All three images show a nearly horizontal wide line of reduced signal intensity in the proximal medial tibia close to the level of the epiphyseal line. Oblique contour disruption of inferior surface of medial meniscal posterior horn

d Sagittal T2*: Horizontal line of increased signal intensity in the proximal tibia (*arrow*). Anterior portion of medial meniscal posterior horn deformed and of abnormally increased signal intensity

Fig. 7.21 a, b. Signs of tibial pseudarthrosis of proximal third following trauma 2 months earlier, no radiograph (71-year-old female)

a Sagittal T1: Discontinuity in proximal third of tibia with local signal decrease. Fracture cleft margin partly surrounded by black margin with anterior and posterior contour bulging. Bridging callus starting to form posteriorly

b Sagittal T2*: Fracture cleft moderately hyperintense – margins in part black and showing pronounced contour bulging. Slight reaction of adjacent muscle/subcutaneous structures

Fig. 7.22 a, b. Posttraumatic osteonecrosis of posterior margin of lateral condyle following distortion 3 months earlier (50-year-old male)

a Sagittal T1: Curved subchondral area of decreased signal intensity in posterior margin of lateral condyle without cortical disruption or chondral involvement

b Sagittal T2*: Subchondral area markedly increased in signal intensity and surrounded by nearly black margin

Fig. 7.23 a, b. Extensive posttraumatic osteonecrosis following rotation injury with tear of lateral meniscal posterior horn 5 months earlier (54-year-old male)

a Sagittal T1: Extensive signal decrease in posterior lateral condyle with subchondral curved portions of slightly higher signal intensity. No cortical disruption or chondral involvement. Possibly contour disruption of lateral meniscal posterior horn

b Sagittal T2*: Pronounced subchondral increase in signal intensity at posterior margin of lateral condyle with only mild hyperintensity of surrounding area. Delicate contour disruptions of lateral meniscal posterior horn, more conspicuous than on the T1-weighted reference section

a

b

8 Medial Meniscal Lesions

8.1 Technique and Method

Imaging is performed predominantly in coronal and sagittal orientations or using 3D acquisition with radial reconstruction perpendicular to the meniscal segment under investigation. The slice thickness should not exceed 3 mm. Degenerative changes and meniscal tears are best evaluated using T1- and T2-weighted sequences as well as fat suppression.

8.2 Anatomy

The medial meniscus is a C-shaped disc of fibrocartilage and is more truly crescent-shaped than the nearly circular lateral meniscus. Both horns of the medial meniscus attach to the intercondylar region anteriorly and posteriorly; these insertion areas are farther apart than those of the lateral meniscus, which lie in between.

The two menisci may be connected at their anterior edges by a transverse ligament. Seen from the side, the medial meniscus is wedge-shaped with the posterior horn being thicker than the mid-portion and the anterior horn.

The outer edge of the meniscus is thickened and connected to the synovial membrane. The major portion of the meniscus is avascular with only the outer one fifth to one third being vascularized in adults.

The medial collateral ligament is embedded in the joint capsule, its deep layers being thereby firmly attached to the medial meniscus.

8.3 Normal MRI Appearance

T1- and T2-weighted images depict the normal meniscus as a homogeneously hypointense to black structure with a central bundle of vessels and nerves of higher signal intensity at the base. The surface is smooth throughout with sharply defined contours. The free edge of the meniscus is acutely angled.

8.4 Pathomechanism

- Isolated traumatic injury of the medial meniscus (rather rare) – forced rotation of the thigh on the loaded and fixed lower leg with the knee flexed.
- Concomitant traumatic injury of the meniscus (fractures around the knee, complex capsuloligamentous lesions).
- Secondary rupture associated with meniscal degeneration.

8.5 Pathophysiology

The following types of meniscal tears are distinguished morphologically (according to *Trillat*):

- Initial tears (longitudinal tears of posterior horn).
- Flap tears.
- Bucket-handle tears.
- Horizontal tears of posterior horn.

The preliminary clinical diagnosis of a meniscal tear is made by eliciting meniscal signs (pain induced by pressing, pulling, and shearing of the different portions of the meniscus) or by demonstrating impingement phenomena. Most acute meniscal injuries are also associated with effusion.

8.6 MRI Signs of Abnormal Findings

Grading

Grade I: *Discreet central degeneration* – demonstration of an intrameniscal lesion of increased signal intensity without connection to articular surface (Fig. 8.1).

Grade II: *Extensive central degeneration* – larger intrameniscal area of increased signal intensity, may be horizontal in orientation or linear, again without connection to articular surface (Figs. 8.2 and 8.3).

Grade III: *Meniscal tear* – increased intrameniscal signal intensity with contour disruption of articular surface, may be associated with displacement of meniscal fragments or superficial step formation (Figs. 8.4–8.9, 8.13).

Grade IV: *Complex meniscal tear* – multiple disruption of meniscal surfaces (Figs. 8.10–8.12, 8.14–8.16).

The main challenge for MRI is the assessment of the meniscal surfaces. The following *rule of thumb* applies:

- No tear without clear-cut connection to surface.
- "Single-slice rule": Extension of abnormal intrameniscal signal to surface on one slice only → inconclusive finding (50% probability of tear).
- Specificity increases to 90% when there are 2 or more abnormal slices.

Orientation of Tears

- Horizontal (Figs. 8.6 and 8.7).
- Vertical (Fig. 8.13).
- Oblique (Figs. 8.4, 8.5, and 8.9).
- Complex tear with several orientations (Figs. 8.10–8.12).

Types of Tears

- Bucket-handle tear, may be associated with displacement toward posterior cruciate ligament ("double-cruciate sign") or with anterior displacement in case of fragmentation ("double-peak sign"; Figs. 8.14–8.16).
- Radial tear (vertical split tear; Fig. 8.13).
- Peripheral tear.
- Tear of discoid meniscus (Fig. 8.5).

A *discoid meniscus* is a congenital deformity that is typically thicker and broader than a normal meniscus (depicted as a continuous structure on more than 2 contiguous 4–5 mm sagittal slices), resulting in a mechanical constellation that makes this variant more susceptible to rupture. Medial discoid menisci (frequency: 0.12–0.3%) are about 10 times less common than lateral discoid menisci (frequency: 1.5–1.6%).

Complications of Meniscal Tears

- Displacement, in particular with bucket-handle tears (Figs. 8.14–8.16).
- Meniscoligamentous separation (distance between meniscal periphery and capsular structures increased to 0.8–1 cm).
- Formation of ganglion cysts (10 times less frequent with medial meniscal tears than with lateral meniscal tears) – circumscribed cystic lesions communicating with the tear. Hyperintense on T2-weighted images. Medical meniscal cysts typically located in the posterior recess of the meniscus (Figs. 8.18 and 8.19).

Postoperative Menisci

Fibrocartilaginous repair mechanisms produce irregular increases in signal intensity along the cut surfaces of partially excised menisci that are difficult to distinguish from residual or new tears.

Moreover, partially resected menisci may contain residual tears that should not be excised further in order to avoid impairing mechanical stability.

8.7 MRI Pitfalls in Medial Meniscal Lesions

Meniscal agenesis (differential diagnosis: meniscectomy or displaced bucket-handle tear) or hypoplasia (Figs. 8.20–8.23). Central intrameniscal vessels in children do not represent degeneration.

8.8 Clinical Role of MRI Findings

Because not all meniscal lesions demonstrated by MRI require invasive treatment, therapeutic decisions should never be based on positive MRI findings alone but must always include the clinical presentation as well.

The demonstration of meniscal lesions by MRI has a crucial role in patients with combined injuries as the menisci, in addition to improving articular congruence, also have stabilizing functions in conjunction with the capsuloligamentous structures.

The differentiation of tears in the red (vascularized) and in the white (avascular) zone of the meniscus is important since reattachment of meniscal fragments is promising only in the vascularized area.

In patients having undergone partial meniscectomy, residual and new tears can be differentiated only by comparison with MR images obtained immediately after surgery.

The clinical relevance of postoperative MRI findings demonstrating intrameniscal lesions is controversial since such abnormal meniscal portions must often be left in place in order to preserve peripheral static stability (Fig. 8.21).

Further Reading

Anderson MW, Raghavan N, Seidenwurm DJ, Greenspan A, Drake C (1995) Evaluation of meniscal tears: fast spin-echo versus conventional spin-echo magnetic resonance imaging. Acad Radiol 2 (3): 209–214

Arkel van ER, Goei R, de Ploeg I, de Boer HH (2000) Meniscal allografts: evaluation with magnetic resonance imaging and correlation with arthroscopy. Arthroscopy 16 (5): 517–521

Blair TR, Schweitzer M, Resnick D (1999) Meniscal cysts causing bone erosion: retrospective analysis of seven cases. Clin Imaging 23 (2): 134–138

Bohnsack M, Ruhmann O, Sander Beuermann A, Wirth CJ (1999) Vergleich der klinischen Untersuchung mit der kernspintomographischen Untersuchung zur Diagnostik von Meniskusläsionen in der täglichen Praxis. Z Orthop Ihre Grenzgeb 137(1):38–42

Cheung LP, Li KC, Hollett MD, Bergman AG, Herfkens RJ (1997) Meniscal tears of the knee: accuracy of detection with fast spin-echo MR imaging and arthroscopic correlation in 293 patients. Radiology 203 (2): 508–512

Connolly B, Babyn PS, Wright JG, Thorner PS (1996) Discoid meniscus in children: magnetic resonance imaging characteristics. Can Assoc Radiol J 47 (5): 347–354

Elvenes J, Jerome CP, Reikeras O, Johansen O (2000) Magnetic resonance imaging as a screening procedure to avoid arthroscopy for meniscal tears. Arch Orthop Trauma Surg 120(1–2):14–16

Horton LK, Jacobson JA, Lin J, Hayes CW (2000) Characterization of the "red zone" of knee meniscus: MR imaging and histologic correlation. Radiology 217 (1): 193–200

Lecas LK, Helms CA, Kosarek FJ, Garret WE (1999) Inferiorly displaced flap tears of the medial meniscus: MR appearance and clinical significance. J Biomech Eng 121(6):161–164

Table 8.1. Characteristic signal intensities

	T1w	T2w	T2*w	rho-w	FAT-SAT
Meniscus	0	0	0	0	0
Central meniscal degeneration	↑	↑ – ↑↑	↑ – ↑↑	↑	↑↑
Meniscal tear	↑	↑ – ↑↑	↑ – ↑↑	↑	↑↑ – ↑↑↑
Meniscal repair zones	↑	↑	↑	↑	↑↑

0 No signal; ↑ low SI; ↑↑ intermediate SI; ↑↑↑ high SI.

Lektrakul N, Skaf A, Yeh L, Roger B, Schweitzer M, Blasbalg R, Resnick D (1999) Pericruciate meniscal cysts arising form tears of the posterior horn of the medial meniscus: MR imaging features that simulate posterior cruciate ganglion cysts. AJR Am J Roentgenol 172 (6): 1575–1579

Lim PS, Schweitzer ME, Bhatia M et al. (1999) Repeat tear of postoperative meniscus: potential MR imaging signs. Radiology 210 (1): 183–188

Ludman CN, Hough DO, Cooper TG, Gottschalk A (1999) Silent meniscal abnormalities in athletes: magnetic resonance imaging of asymptomatic competitive gymnasts. Br J Sports Med 33 (6): 414–416

Magee TH, Hinson GW (1998) MRI of meniscal bucket-handle tears. Skeletal Radiol 27 (9): 495–499

Muellner T, Nikolic A, Kubiena H, Kainberger F, Mettlboeck M, Vecsei V (1999) The role of magnetic resonance imaging in routine decision making for meniscal surgery. Knee Surg Sports Traumatol Arthrosc 7 (5): 278–283

Muellner T, Weinstabl R, Schabus R, Vecsei V, Kainberger F (1997) The diagnosis of meniscal tears in athletes. A comparison of clinical and magnetic resonance imaging investigations. Am J Sports Med 25 (1): 7–12

Nawata K, Teshima R, Enokida M, Suzuki T, Yamagata T (1999) Magnetic resonance imaging of meniscal degeneration in torn menisci: a comparison between anterior cruciate ligament deficient knees and stable knees. Knee Surg Sports Traumatol Arthrosc 7 (5): 274–277

Rappeport ED, Wieslander SB, Stephensen S, Lausten GS, Thomsen HS (1997) MRI preferable to diagnostic arthroscopy in knee joint injuries. A double-blind comparison of 47 patients. Acta Orthop Scand 68 (3): 277–281

Rubin DA (1997) MR imaging of the knee menisci. Radiol Clin North Am 35(1):21–44

Rubin DA, Paletta GA Jr (2000) Current concepts and controversies in meniscal imaging. Magn Reson Imaging Clin N Am 8(2):243–270

Schaefer WD, Martin DF, Pope TL Jr, Rudicil HS (1996) Meniscal ossicle. J South Orthop Assoc 5 (2): 126–129

Sciulli RL, Boutin RD, Brown RR et al. (1999) Evaluation of the postoperative meniscus of the knee: a study comparing conventional arthrography, conventional MR imaging, MR arthrography with iodinated contrast material, and MR arthrography with gadolinium-based contrast material. Skeletal Radiol 28 (9): 508–514

Tasker AD, Ostlere SJ (1995) Relative incidence and morphology of lateral and medial meniscal cysts detected by magnetic resonance imaging. Clin Radiol 50 (11): 778–781

Totty WG, Matava MJ (2000) Imaging the postoperative meniscus. Magn Reson Imaging Clin N Am 8 (2): 271–283

Trillat A (1962) Lesions traumatique du menisque interne du genou. Classement anatomique et diagnostic clinique. Rev Chir Orthop 48: 551

Tuite MJ, De Smet AA, Swan JS, Keene JS (1995) MR imaging of a meniscal ossicle. Skeletal Radiol 24 (7): 543–545

Tyson LL, Daughters TC Jr, Ryu RK, Crues JV III (1995) MRI appearance of meniscal cysts. Skeletal Radiol 24 (6): 421–424

Uppal A, Disler DG, Short WB, McCauley TR, Cooper JA (1998) Internal derangements of the knee: rates of occurrence at MR imaging in patients referred by orthopedic surgeons compared with rates in patients referred by physicians who are not orthopedic surgeons. Radiology 207 (3): 633–636

Watt AJ, Halliday T, Raby N (2000) The value of the absent bow tie sign in MRI of bucket-handle tears. Clin Radiol 55 (8): 622–626

White LM, Schweitzer ME, Johnson WJ, Amster BJ, Oliveri MP, Russell K (1996) The role of T2-weighted fast-spin-echo imaging in the diagnosis of meniscal tears. J Magn Reson Imaging 6 (6): 874–877

Wright DH, De Smet AA, Norris M (1995) Bucket-handle tears of the medial and lateral menisci of the knee: value of MR imaging in detecting displaced fragments. AJR Am J Roentgenol 165 (3): 621–625

Fig. 8.1 a, b. Central degeneration of medial meniscal posterior horn, grade I (23-year-old female)

a Sagittal T1; **b** sagittal T2*: Slight central increase in signal intensity in posterior horn of medial meniscus without contour disruption

a

b

Fig. 8.2 a, b. Central degeneration of medial meniscal posterior horn, grade II (36-year-old male)

a Sagittal T1; b sagittal T2*: More extensive central increase in signal intensity in posterior horn of medial meniscus extending in the direction of the inferior surface but without contour disruption (borderline tear)

a

b

Fig. 8.3 a, b. Central degeneration of medial meniscal posterior horn, grade II (29-year-old male)

a Sagittal T1; **b** sagittal T2*: Extensive, partly linear, signal increase in posterior horn of medial meniscus without contour disruption

Fig. 8.4. Very discreet tear of medial meniscal posterior horn, inferior surface, initial grade III tear (55-year-old female)

Coronal T1: Discreet increase in intrameniscal signal intensity with barely discernible contour disruption of inferior surface (*arrow*)

Fig. 8.5 a, b. Discreet tear of medial meniscal posterior horn, grade III, medial discoid meniscus (41-year-old male)

a Coronal T1: Slight contour disruption of inferior surface of peripheral part of medial meniscus (*arrow*). Slight central signal increase in lateral third (*arrowhead*)

b Sagittal T2*: Discreet contour disruption of inferior surface (*arrow*). Discoid meniscus with continuity of anterior and posterior horns on more than 2 slices (*not shown*)

a

b

Fig. 8.6a, b. Tear of medial meniscal posterior horn at transition to midportion, grade III (63-year-old male)

a Coronal T1: Horizontal contour disruption of superior surface of posterior horn of medial meniscus (*arrow*)

b Sagittal T2*: Pronounced horizontal increase in signal intensity in posterior horn with contour disruption of superior surface

Fig. 8.7 a, b. Horizontal tear of medial meniscal posterior horn, grade III (17-year-old male)

a Coronal T1; **b** sagittal T2*: Both images show horizontally oriented, extended contour disruption of superior surface of posterior horn of medial meniscus (*arrows*)

a

b

Fig. 8.8a, b. Extensive tear of medial meniscal posterior horn, grade III (38-year-old male)

a Coronal T1: Extensive increase in intrameniscal signal intensity in posterior horn of medial meniscus with contour disruption of superior surface (*arrow*)

b Sagittal T2*: Considerable increase in intrameniscal signal with contour disruption of superior surface (*arrow*) and thinning of inferior surface (*arrowhead*)

a

b

Fig. 8.9 a, b. Extensive tear of medial meniscal posterior horn, grade III (36-year-old male)

a Sagittal T1; **b** sagittal T2*: Sharply demarcated linear signal increase, slightly undulated posteriorly, in posterior horn of medial meniscus with contour disruption of inferior surface

a

b

Fig. 8.10. Complex tear of medial meniscal posterior horn, grade IV (39-year-old male)

Sagittal T2*: Linear signal increase in posterior horn of medial meniscus with contour disruptions of superior and inferior surfaces (*arrow*)

Fig. 8.11 a, b. Complex tear of medial meniscal posterior horn, grade IV (28-year-old male)

a Sagittal T1; **b** sagittal T2*: Linear intrameniscal signal increase with broad contour disruption of inferior surface and delicate contour disruption of superior surface (*arrows*)

ⓐ

ⓑ

Fig. 8.12 a, b. Complex tear of medial meniscal posterior horn, grade IV (54-year-old male)

a Sagittal T1; **b** sagittal T2*: Pronounced contour disruptions of superior and inferior surfaces of posterior horn of medial meniscus with central linear increases in intrameniscal signal on both sequences. Joint effusion

a

b

Fig. 8.13 a, b. Vertical tear of medial meniscal posterior horn, grade III, discoid meniscus (47-year-old male)

a Coronal T1: Extremely thick posterior horn with vertical discontinuity in peripheral quarter of medial meniscus (*arrow*)

b Sagittal T2*: Vertical contour disruption of posterior horn at transition to midportion. Continuity of anterior and posterior horns on more than 2 sagittal slices (adjacent slices *not shown*)

a

b

c

d

Fig. 8.14a–d. Displaced bucket-handle tear of medial meniscus (19-year-old male)

a Coronal T1: Vertical contour disruption of posterior horn of medial meniscus, lateral third (*arrow*). Additional horizontally oriented linear increase in intrameniscal signal intensity with contour disruption of inferior surface in central and peripheral segments

b Coronal T1: Meniscal continuity disrupted over extended area: fragments displaced peripherally and toward the margin of eminence (*arrows*)

c Sagittal T2*: Truncated appearance of posterior horn with additional linear increase in signal intensity and contour disruption (*arrow*)

d Sagittal T2*: Large part of the midportion/previous free margin displaced toward eminence, where it is seen as an intermediate-signal-intensity band with irregular contours (*arrow*)

a

b

c

d

Fig. 8.15a–d. Displaced fragmented bucket-handle tear of medial meniscus (18-year-old male)

a Coronal T1: Posterior medial meniscal recess mostly empty except for some faintly discernible medial and peripheral meniscal remnants

b Coronal T1: Large portion of medial meniscus displaced toward eminence where it appears as an "upside-down V" (*arrow*)

c Sagittal T1: Empty posterior meniscal recess, except for obliquely sectioned local fat of hyperintense signal. Abnormally thickened part of anterior horn with markedly increased signal intensity basally (*arrow*)

d Sagittal T1: Part of medial meniscus appearing as a band displaced toward eminence (*arrow*)

a

b

c

d

Fig. 8.16a–d. Displaced bucket-handle tear of medial meniscus (60-year-old male)

a, b Coronal T1: Contour of posterior horn of medial meniscus disrupted in middle third with displacement of larger portions toward eminence (*arrows*)

c Sagittal T1; **d** sagittal T2*: Parts of anterior horn not clearly discernible. Abnormal contour doubling of posterior horn produced by displaced parts (*arrows*)

Fig. 8.17a–c. Small ossification at medial meniscal posterior horn; discreet tear of inferior surface (21-year-old male)

a Coronal T1: Circular hyperintense structure (equivalent to fat/bone) at the free margin of the posterior horn of the medial meniscus (*arrow*)

b Sagittal T1: Shortened posterior horn with a triangular hyperintensity in the cranial half (*arrow*) obscuring directly adjacent tear of inferior surface (cf. **c**)

c Sagittal T2*: Abnormal calcification depicted on T1-weighting (**a, b**) no longer seen. Instead, delicate contour disruption of inferior surface more clearly discernible (*arrow*)

Fig. 8.18a, b. Ganglion cyst of medial meniscus (15-year-old female)

a Coronal T1; **b** coronal T2*: Ovoid to triangular distention of peripheral medial meniscal posterior horn and circumscribed cystic lesion isointense to fluid (*arrows*)

a

b

a

b

c

d

Fig. 8.19a–d. Extensive ganglion cyst of medial meniscus/capsule, grade III posterior horn tear (38-year-old female)

a Coronal T1: Ovoid capsular cystic lesion (nearly isointense to muscle) in medial compartment. In addition, peripheral intrameniscal signal increase in medial meniscal posterior horn (*arrow*)

b Axial T2*: Hyperintense fluid collection with partial septation at the medial margin of the joint capsule

c, d Sagittal T2*: Slightly flattened medial meniscal posterior horn with linear contour disruption of inferior surface (*arrow* in **c**). In addition, delicate connection from the medial meniscal posterior recess (**c**) to a large, markedly hyperintense cystic fluid collection with partial septation and extracapsular extension

Fig. 8.20 a, b. Status post arthroscopic partial meniscectomy (25-year-old male)

a Coronal T1: Circumscribed defect of inferior surface of posterior horn of medial meniscus (*arrow*)

b Sagittal T1: Anterior base of medial meniscal posterior horn appears to be partly truncated (*arrow*)

a

b

a

b

c

d

Fig. 8.21 a – d. Residual/new tear of medial meniscal posterior horn following arthroscopic partial meniscectomy $^1/_2$ year earlier – no repeat intervention (15-year-old female)

a Coronal T1: Irregular residual structures of posterior horn of medial meniscus with contour disruptions (*arrow*)

b Sagittal T1: Irregularities and contour defects at the posterior horn/midportion junction (*arrow*)

c, d Sagittal T1: Obliquely oriented contour disruption of inferior surface of residual posterior horn (*arrows*). Note: Excision of the inferior surface leaving behind a residual horizontal or oblique tear near the base may suggest a normal postoperative status at MRI, especially since MRI frequently cannot identify regenerative cartilage

Fig. 8.22 a, b. Irregularities/persisting tears of medial meniscus/regenerative cartilage formation following 2 partial meniscectomies 3 and 2 years earlier (25-year-old female)

a Sagittal T1; **b** sagittal T2*: Irregular residual structures in the recess of the posterior horn; poorly visualized on T1-weighting, more clearly appreciated on relatively T2-weighted image (*arrow*)

a

b

Fig. 8.23 a, b. Displaced residual medial meniscal posterior horn/ regenerative cartilage formation following partial meniscectomy $^1/_2$ year earlier (49-year-old female)

a Coronal T1: Curved isolated structure of meniscal signal intensity at lateral margin of medial condyle (*arrow*)

b Axial T2*: Ovoid low-signal-intensity remnants of meniscus in paramedian location at posterior margin of medial condyle (*arrow*)

a

b

9 Lateral Meniscal Lesions

9.1 Technique and Method

Imaging of the lateral meniscus is performed in the same way as assessment of the medial meniscus.

9.2 Anatomy

The lateral meniscus forms an almost closed ring. Like the medial meniscus, it also inserts anteriorly and posteriorly into the intercondylar area, between the insertion sites of the medial meniscus.

The lateral meniscus has a fairly loose bond to the joint capsule and is not connected with the lateral collateral ligament, which itself is separated from the joint capsule by a cleft. The tendon of the popliteal muscle courses freely in the joint capsule and it is in this area that the posterior horn of the lateral meniscus is free. The posterior end of the lateral meniscus may have ligamentous attachments to the medial femoral condyle (anterior and posterior meniscofemoral ligaments).

9.3 Normal MRI Appearance

While the medial meniscus has a prominent posterior horn and is semilunar in shape, the lateral meniscus is more circular in configuration and altogether more symmetrical with an anterior and a posterior horn of nearly identical height (Fig. 9.1).

Like the medial meniscus, the lateral meniscus appears hypointense in all sequences. Medial portions of the anterior horn of the lateral meniscus show slight spreading of fibers. Another specific feature of the lateral meniscus is its loose synovial connection to the popliteal tendon in the area of the posterior horn. There is no direct anatomic connection between the lateral meniscus and the lateral collateral ligament.

9.4 Pathomechanism

Lesions of the lateral meniscus are much less common than lesions of the medial meniscus (1:20) and may occur in connection with complex injuries or on the basis of meniscal degeneration.

9.5 MRI Signs of Abnormal Findings

Grading

Abnormalities of the lateral meniscus are graded in the same way as medial meniscal lesions.

Grade I: *Discreet central degeneration* – demonstration of an intrameniscal lesion of increased signal intensity without connection to articular surface.

Grade II: *Extensive central degeneration* – larger intrameniscal area of increased signal intensity, may be horizontal in orientation or linear, again without connection to articular surface (Fig. 9.4).

Grade III: *Meniscal tear* – increased intrameniscal signal intensity with contour disruption of articular surface, may be associated with displacement of meniscal fragments or superficial step formation (Figs. 9.5–9.9).

Grade IV: Complex meniscal tear – multiple disruption of meniscal surfaces (Figs. 9.10–9.18).

Types of Tears

The types of meniscal tears that may occur are in principle the same for both menisci (see Chap. 8). However, lesions of the anterior horn, because it is stronger laterally, are more common in the lateral meniscus. Bucket-handle tears, on the other hand, predominantly occur medially, and ruptures in the area of the base with meniscocapsular separation exclusively affect the medial meniscus.

Discoid Meniscus

This congenital meniscal deformity is 10 times more common laterally than medially (incidence of 1.5–1.6% and 0.12–0.3%, respectively). The unfavorable mechanical constellation makes discoid menisci more prone to rupture (Figs. 9.15, 9.17, 9.23–9.26).

Complications of Meniscal Tears

Ganglion cysts associated with torn menisci are 10 times more common in the lateral meniscus than in the medial meniscus. They are depicted on T2-weighted images as hyperintense circumscribed fluid collections that communicate with the tear. Lateral ganglion cysts more commonly occur in the area of the base, mostly with anterior extension toward Hoffa's fat pad (Figs. 9.19–9.22; see also Fig. 11.14).

9.6 MRI Pitfalls in Assessing the Lateral Meniscus

- Oblique sectioning of anterior transverse meniscal ligament of Winslow at anterior horn (Fig. 9.3).
- Oblique sectioning of Wrisberg's ligament at posterior horn.
- Fat layer separating posterior horn from popliteal tendon (Fig. 9.2).
- Central myxoid degeneration or marginal fibrillation (Fig. 9.4).
- Small menisci (status post partial meniscectomy, arthritis, bucket-handle tear, hypoplasia).
- Fenestration of discoid menisci.

9.7 Clinical Role of MRI Findings

What has been said for the medial meniscus also applies to the lateral meniscus (see Chap. 8). In terms of topographic anatomy, the examiner must be aware of the popliteal hiatus, which must not be mistaken for a meniscal tear and, accordingly, must not be closed when meniscal repair is performed.

Table 9.1. Characteristic signal intensities

	T1w	T2w	T2*w	rho-w	FAT-SAT
Meniscus	0	0	0	0	0
Central meniscal degeneration	↑	↑ – ↑↑	↑ – ↑↑	↑	↑↑
Meniscal tear	↑	↑ – ↑↑	↑ – ↑↑	↑	↑↑ – ↑↑↑
Meniscal repair zones	↑	↑	↑	↑	↑↑

0 No signal; ↑ low SI; ↑↑ intermediate SI; ↑↑↑ high SI.

Further Reading

Anderson MW, Raghavan N, Seidenwurm DJ, Greenspan A, Drake C (1995) Evaluation of meniscal tears: fast spin-echo versus conventional spin-echo magnetic resonance imaging. Acad Radiol 2 (3): 209–214

Araki Y, Ashikaga R, Fujii K, Ishida O, Hamada M, Ueda J, Tsukaguchi I (1998) MR imaging of meniscal tears with discoid lateral meniscus. Eur J Radiol 27 (2): 153–160

Arkel van ER, Goei R, de Ploeg I, de Boer HH (2000) Meniscal allografts: evaluation with magnetic resonance imaging and correlation with arthroscopy. Arthroscopy 16 (5): 517–521

Blair TR, Schweitzer M, Resnick D (1999) Meniscal cysts causing bone erosion: retrospective analysis of seven cases. Clin Imaging 23 (2): 134–138

Bohnsack M, Ruhmann O, Sander Beuermann A, Wirth CJ (1999) Vergleich der klinischen Untersuchung mit der kernspintomographischen Untersuchung zur Diagnostik von Meniskusläsionen in der täglichen Praxis. Z Orthop Ihre Grenzgeb 137 (1): 38–42

Cheung LP, Li KC, Hollett MD, Bergman AG, Herfkens RJ (1997) Meniscal tears of the knee: accuracy of detection with fast spin-echo MR imaging and arthroscopic correlation in 293 patients. Radiology 203 (2): 508–512

Connolly B, Babyn PS, Wright JG, Thorner PS (1996) Discoid meniscus in children: magnetic resonance imaging characteristics. Can Assoc Radiol J 47 (5): 347–354

Elvenes J, Jerome CP, Reikeras O, Johansen O (2000) Magnetic resonance imaging as a screening procedure to avoid arthroscopy for meniscal tears. Arch Orthop Trauma Surg 120 (1–2): 14–16

Horton LK, Jacobson JA, Lin-J, Hayes CW (2000) Characterization of the "red zone" of knee meniscus: MR imaging and histologic correlation. Radiology 217 (1): 193–200

Lim PS, Schweitzer ME, Bhatia M et al. (1999) Repeat tear of postoperative meniscus: potential MR imaging signs. Radiology 210 (1): 183–188

Ludman CN, Hough DO, Cooper TG, Gottschalk A (1999) Silent meniscal abnormalities in athletes: magnetic resonance imaging of asymptomatic competitive gymnasts. Br J Sports Med 33 (6): 414–416

Magee TH, Hinson GW (1998) MRI of meniscal bucket-handle tears. Skeletal Radiol 27 (9): 495–499

Muellner T, Nikolic A, Kubiena H, Kainberger F, Mettlboeck M, Vecsei V (1999) The role of magnetic resonance imaging in routine decision making for meniscal surgery. Knee Surg Sports Traumatol Arthrosc 7 (5): 278–283

Muellner T, Weinstabl R, Schabus R, Vecsei V, Kainberger F (1997) The diagnosis of meniscal tears in athletes. A comparison of clinical and magnetic resonance imaging investigations. Am J Sports Med 25 (1): 7–12

Nawata K, Teshima R, Enokida M, Suzuki T, Yamagata T (1999) Magnetic resonance imaging of meniscal degeneration in torn menisci: a comparison between anterior cruciate ligament deficient knees and stable knees. Knee Surg Sports Traumatol Arthrosc 7 (5): 274–277

Rappeport ED, Wieslander SB, Stephensen S, Lausten GS, Thomsen HS (1997) MRI preferable to diagnostic arthroscopy in knee joint injuries. A double-blind comparison of 47 patients. Acta Orthop Scand 68 (3): 277–281

Rubin DA (1997) MR imaging of the knee menisci. Radiol Clin North Am 35 (1): 21–44

Rubin DA, Paletta GA Jr (2000) Current concepts and controversies in meniscal imaging. Magn Reson Imaging Clin N Am 8 (2): 243–270

Ryu KN, Kim IS, Kim EJ, Ahn JW, Bae DK, Sartoris DJ, Resnick D (1998) MR imaging of tears of discoid lateral menisci. AJR Am J Roentgenol 171 (4): 963–967

Schaefer WD, Martin DF, Pope TL Jr, Rudicil HS (1996) Meniscal ossicle. J South Orthop Assoc 5 (2): 126–129

Sciulli RL, Boutin RD, Brown RR et al. (1999) Evaluation of the postoperative meniscus of the knee: a study comparing conventional arthrography, conventional MR imaging, MR arthrography with iodinated contrast material, and MR arthrography with gadolinium-based contrast material. Skeletal Radiol 28 (9): 508–514

Shankman S, Beltran J, Melamed E, Rosenberg ZS (1997) Anterior horn of the lateral meniscus: another potential pitfall in MR imaging of the knee. Radiology 204 (1): 181–184

Tasker AD, Ostlere SJ (1995) Relative incidence and morphology of lateral and medial meniscal cysts detected by magnetic resonance imaging. Clin Radiol 50 (11): 778–781

Totty WG, Matava MJ (2000) Imaging the postoperative meniscus. Magn Reson Imaging Clin N Am 8 (2): 271–283

Tuite MJ, De Smet AA, Swan JS, Keene JS (1995) MR imaging of a meniscal ossicle. Skeletal Radiol 24 (7): 543–545

Tyson LL, Daughters TC Jr, Ryu RK, Crues JV III (1995) MRI appearance of meniscal cysts. Skeletal Radiol 24 (6): 421–424

Uppal A, Disler DG, Short WB, McCauley TR, Cooper JA (1998) Internal derangements of the knee: rates of occurrence at MR imaging in patients referred by orthopedic surgeons compared with rates in patients referred by physicians who are not orthopedic surgeons. Radiology 207 (3): 633–636

Watt AJ, Halliday T, Raby N (2000) The value of the absent bow tie sign in MRI of bucket-handle tears. Clin Radiol 55 (8): 622–626

White LM, Schweitzer ME, Johnson WJ, Amster BJ, Oliveri MP, Russell K (1996) The role of T2-weighted fast-spin-echo imaging in the diagnosis of meniscal tears. J Magn Reson Imaging 6 (6): 874–877

Wright DH, De Smet AA, Norris M (1995) Bucket-handle tears of the medial and lateral menisci of the knee: value of MR imaging in detecting displaced fragments. AJR Am J Roentgenol 165 (3): 621–625

Fig. 9.1. Normal lateral meniscus (20-year-old female)

Sagittal; *left* T1, *right* T2*: Lateral meniscus depicted as a homogeneous structure of absent signal intensity in both sequences. Good delineation of popliteal compartment on T1-weighting (*left image*)

Fig. 9.2 a, b. Pseudotear of lateral meniscus: oblique sectioning of posterior meniscal ligament (23-year-old male)

a, b Sagittal T1: Square to rectangular structure posterior to lateral meniscal posterior horn, separated from meniscus by a delicate line (*arrows*) – no meniscal tear

a

b

Fig. 9.3 a, b. Pseudotear of lateral meniscus: oblique sectioning of meniscal ligaments (48-year-old female)

a, b Sagittal T1: Delicate lines of brighter signal separating anterior and posterior horns from directly adjacent meniscal ligaments (*arrows*)

a

b

a

b

Fig. 9.4 a, b. Predominant central degeneration of lateral meniscal posterior horn; fissuring of inferior surface, grade II – III (30-year-old male)

a Coronal T1: Definite roundish area of increased signal intensity with linear peripheral extension in posterior horn of lateral meniscus (*arrow*)

b Sagittal T1: Area of increased intrameniscal signal in part close to inferior surface. Thinning of base part. Images provide no evidence of contour disruption

Fig. 9.5 a, b. Delicate partial tear of lateral meniscal posterior horn, grade III (33-year-old female)

a Sagittal T1; **b** sagittal T2*: Discreet triangular incongruity of inferior surface with locally increased signal intensity in both sequences (*arrows*)

a

b

Fig. 9.6. Tear of lateral meniscal posterior horn, grade III (14-year-old girl)

Sagittal T2*: Obliquely oriented line of increased signal intensity through posterior horn of lateral meniscus with contour disruption of inferior surface (*arrow*)

a

b

Fig. 9.7 a, b. Horizontal tear of lateral meniscal posterior horn, grade III (37-year-old male)

a Coronal T1: Linear increase in signal intensity in posterior horn of lateral meniscus with contour disruption of posterior surface (*arrow*)

b Sagittal T2*: Horizontal contour disruption of posterior horn of lateral meniscus (*arrow*)

Fig. 9.8 a, b. Tear of lateral meniscal anterior horn, grade III (26-year-old male)

a Coronal T1: Wedge-shaped contour disruption of anterior horn of lateral meniscus (*arrow*) – body of meniscus abnormally thickened by displaced portion

b Sagittal T2*: Curved and partly horizontal line of increased signal intensity consistent with contour disruption of lateral meniscal anterior horn (*arrow*)

Fig. 9.9 a, b. Tear of lateral meniscal anterior horn, grade III (59-year-old female)

a Sagittal T1; **b** sagittal T2*: Both images show horizontal line of increased signal intensity and contour defects of lateral meniscal anterior horn, most conspicuous on relatively T2-weighted image (**b**)

a

b

c

d

Fig. 9.10a–d. Displaced, fragmented bucket-handle tear (33-year-old male)

a Coronal T1: Abnormally thickened parts of posterior horn of lateral meniscus displaced medially (*arrow*)

b Axial T2*: Larger posteromedial fragment of lateral meniscus depicted as a curved band in the area of the intercondylar fossa medial to lateral condyle (*arrow*). Small isolated fragment lateral to posterior parts of lateral condyle (*arrowhead*)

c Sagittal T1; d sagittal T2*: Large curved fragment of lateral meniscus showing mild central hyperintensity on both sequences displaced in the direction of eminence (*arrows*)

Fig. 9.11 a, b. Displaced tear of lateral meniscus (55-year-old female)

a Sagittal T2*: Empty posterior meniscal recess, only fluid collection present (*arrow*)

b Sagittal T2*: Larger, longitudinal fragment of lateral meniscus displaced toward eminence (*arrow*)

a

b

Fig. 9.12 a, b. Displaced bucket-handle tear of lateral meniscus (49-year-old male)

a Sagittal T2*: Empty posterior meniscal recess, only hyperintense fluid present (*arrow*). Cystic out-pouching of anterior meniscotibial capsule – differential diagnosis: small fluid collection at posterior margin of Hoffa's fat pad

b Sagittal T2*: Curved, thickened compact parts of lateral meniscus displaced in the direction of eminence (*arrow*). Bowl-shaped defect of tibial plateau suggesting a cyst-like lesion with debris (*arrowhead*)

Fig. 9.13 a, b. Displaced bucket-handle tear of lateral meniscus (43-year-old male)

a Coronal T1: Wide dehiscence of posterior horn of lateral meniscus with lateral displacement of a smaller fragment (*arrowhead*) and medial displacement of a slightly larger fragment in the direction of eminence (*arrow*)

b Sagittal T2*: Empty posterior meniscal recess – only fluid present

a

b

a

b

c

d

Fig. 9.14a–d. Anteriorly displaced, fragmented bucket-handle tear of lateral meniscus – double-peak sign; disturbed tibial ossification with isolated apophyseal ossification center (15-year-old male)

a Coronal T1: Posterior lateral meniscal recess empty except for a small, medially displaced remnant of meniscus (*arrowhead*)

b Coronal T1: Abnormally enlarged portion of lateral meniscal posterior horn with contour disruption (*arrow*)

c Sagittal T1; **d** sagittal T2*: Both images show empty posterior meniscal recess – obliquely sectioned fat of hyperintense signal intensity on T1-weighted image mimics residual meniscus on relative T2-weighting (*arrowheads*). Double-peak sign of anterior horn of lateral meniscus caused by anteriorly displaced parts (*arrows*). Isolated bone element between tuberosity and distal patellar tendon (*open arrow*)

a

b

c

d

Fig. 9.15 a–d. Displaced bucket-handle tear of lateral meniscus, incomplete discoid meniscus; double-peak sign (16-year-old male)

a Coronal T1: Multiple medial and lateral contour disruption of posterior horn of lateral meniscus (*arrowheads*)

b Sagittal T1: Larger parts of lateral meniscus displaced medially toward eminence with continuity between posterior and anterior horn (*arrow*)

c Sagittal T1; d sagittal T2*: Double-peak sign of anterior horn caused by anteriorly displaced parts of lateral meniscus (*arrows*)

Fig. 9.16a, b. Displaced tear of lateral meniscus: double-peak sign of anterior horn (17-year-old male)

a Sagittal T1; **b** sagittal T2*: Posterior horn abnormally flattened compared to anterior horn. In addition, double-peak sign of anterior horn caused by anteriorly displaced parts of lateral meniscus (*arrows*)

a

b

c

d

Fig. 9.17 a–d. Multiple tear of lateral discoid meniscus with partial displacement, double-peak sign of anterior horn (17-year-old male)

a Sagittal T1: Multiple disruption of lateral meniscus with displacement of a triangular fragment to front of anterior horn (*arrow*)

b, c Sagittal T1; **d** sagittal T2*: Lateral meniscus seen in continuity on several sagittal sections – flattened posterior horn; double-peak sign of anterior horn caused by displaced meniscal parts. Discreet bone contusion of lateral condyle with slight subchondral signal decrease on T1-weighting and increased signal on relative T2-weighting without cortical disruption (*arrows*)

Fig. 9.18. Tear of lateral meniscus, midportion/anterior horn, grade III (63-year-old female)

Sagittal T2*: Vertical contour disruption between midportion and thickened anterior horn (*arrow*)

Fig. 9.19. Emerging ganglion cyst of lateral meniscus in the presence of delicate tear of anterior horn/midportion (24-year-old male)

Sagittal T1: Roundish area of increased signal intensity in anterior horn of lateral meniscus (*arrow*). Step formation between anterior horn and midportion with local contour thinning (*arrowhead*)

Fig. 9.20. Ganglion cyst of lateral meniscus (30-year-old female)

Sagittal T2*: Roundish signal increase at anterior margin of anterior horn of lateral meniscus with faintly discernible defect of anterior surface of meniscus

Fig. 9.21 a, b. Large ganglion cyst of lateral meniscus in the presence of tear of anterior horn (not shown) (15-year-old female)

a Sagittal T2*; **b** axial T2*: Partly lobulated, partly septated ovoid cystic lesion with fluid signal directly in front of anterior horn of lateral meniscus within adjacent lateral parts of Hoffa's fat pad

a

b

a

b

c

d

Fig. 9.22 a – d. Ganglion cyst of lateral meniscus in the presence of tear of anterior horn/midportion (32-year-old male)

a Coronal T1: Triangular dehiscence of peripheral lateral meniscus with contiguous ovoid cystic lesion of slightly hyperintense signal intensity on T1-weighted image

b, c Coronal T2*; **d** sagittal T2*: All three images show marked hyperintensity of the cystic lesion at meniscal margin with some septa and extension into peripheral meniscus

a

b

Fig. 9.23 a, b. Lateral discoid meniscus (13-year-old boy)

a Coronal T1; **b** sagittal T1: Lateral meniscus much larger than medial meniscus (*arrows*), depicted in continuity on several sagittal slices (adjacent slices *not shown*)

Fig. 9.24 a, b. Tear of lateral discoid meniscus, midportion/ transition to anterior horn; medial calcification of lateral meniscal posterior horn (55-year-old male)

a Coronal T1: Contour defect of superior surface of lateral quarter of lateral meniscal posterior horn (*arrow*). Roundish area isointense to marrow at posterior free edge of lateral meniscus (*arrowhead*)

b Sagittal T1: Faintly discernible wedge-shaped contour defect of anterior horn/transition to midportion (*arrow*)

a

b

Fig. 9.25. Tear of lateral discoid meniscus/midportion (44-year-old male)

Sagittal T2*: Contour defect of inferior surface at transition of anterior horn/midportion (*arrow*). Abnormal size of lateral meniscus with compact anterior horn

Fig. 9.26 a, b. Multiple tear of lateral discoid meniscus with partial displacement/emerging ganglion cyst (55-year-old female)

a, b Sagittal T2*: Thinning and contour disruptions of midportion at transition to anterior horn (*arrows*). In addition, contour disruptions of anterior surface of anterior horn with beginning cyst formation (*arrowheads*)

a

b

Fig. 9.27 a, b. Calcification of lateral and medial meniscal posterior horns (63-year-old female)

a Coronal T1: Roundish lesions isointense to marrow at medial and lateral posterior margins of lateral meniscus (*arrows*) and at free margin of posterior horn of medial meniscus (*arrowhead*)

b Sagittal T1: Triangular formation isointense to marrow in lateral posterior meniscal recess

a

b

10 Infrapatellar Fat Pad Lesions, Loose Bodies, Prepatellar Bursae

10.1 Technique and Method

Along with T1-weighted imaging, T2-weighted and fat-suppressed sequences are particularly suited to identify lesions within the adipose tissue of Hoffa's fat pad. Additional imaging after intravenous contrast medium administration may be useful in assessing reactive synovial proliferation or tumor-related changes.

10.2 Anatomy

Hoffa's fat pad is a malleable structure lying below the patella between the synovial membrane and the fibrous membrane of the joint capsule where it fills a variable space whose configuration changes with the movement of the joint. The infrapatellar fat pad is wedge-shaped and may continue proximally in three synovial plicae.

The prepatellar bursa may be subcutaneous, subfascial, or subtendinous in location and never has a connection to the joint cavity.

10.3 Normal MRI Appearance

Hoffa's fat pad consists of fatty tissue divided into compartments by fibrous structures. Consequently, its signal is isointense to fat in all sequences, i.e. markedly hyperintense on T1-weighted images, moderately hyperintense on T2-weighted images, and hypointense on relatively T2-weighted images (Fig. 10.1).

The prepatellar and infrapatellar bursae are hypointense on T1-weighted images only in a flat zone extending no more than 0.5 cm in depth and typically do not show much increase in signal on relatively T2-weighted images or fat-suppressed T2-weighted images.

10.4 Pathomechanism/Pathophysiology

- Hoffa's disease – the enlargement of the infrapatellar fat pad by proliferation of fatty tissue – is no longer considered a separate disease entity. Instead, it is now held that it is a condition occurring secondary to other disorders of the knee area.
- Chronic irritation of the knee or overuse may cause symptomatic fibrosis and hyperplasia of a plica, in particular of the medial patellar plica.
- Intra-articular loose bodies occur in articular chondromatosis and severe degenerative joint disease (gonarthrosis) or represent displaced bone fragments detached from the native bone in aseptic bone necrosis and chondral or osteochondral fractures.
- Prepatellar bursitis may be acute or chronic but more important is the distinction of purulent and nonpurulent inflammation of the bursa.

10.5 MRI Signs of Abnormal Findings

Fat Pad Hypertrophy

Fatty tissue proliferation of Hoffa's fat pad most often leads to posterior extension toward the intercondylar fossa and may result in reversible impingement of the protruding parts, seen as hypointensity on T1-weighted images and increased signal intensity at relative T2-weighting (Fig. 10.2).

Fat Pad Tears

Tears of the infrapatellar fat pad are depicted by MRI as disruptions of surface continuity. Fluid having entered the cleft is identified by a reduced signal intensity on T1-weighted images and increased signal on relative and pure T2-weighting. There may be necrosis as a secondary complication (with low or absent signal intensity on all sequences; Figs. 10.3–10.5).

Fat Pad Inflammation (Hoffa'itis)

Inflammation is characterized by a diffuse signal decrease of the fat pad on T1-weighted images and an increased signal intensity on relative T2-weighting. Reactive exudative or proliferative synovial inflammation associated with rheumatoid arthritis may involve the fat pad and is identified on MRI as focal signal changes with otherwise normal signal intensity (Fig. 10.6).

Fat Pad Tumors

Ganglion-like cysts may occur within Hoffa's fat pad as well as circumscribed focal areas of synovial proliferation and synoviomas. These changes appear hyperintense on T2-weighted images. Most ganglion cysts show partial septation. Intravenous administration of a contrast medium is in particular required when assessing synovial proliferation (Figs. 10.7–10.11).

Intra-articular Loose Bodies

Loose bodies in the joint space have low or absent signal intensity in all sequences and can be clearly delineated from hyperintense fluid, especially on T2-weighted images. Such loose bodies comprise articular chondromas, joint osteomas with marrow signal (cf. Figs. 11.2, 11.3, 11.15, and 11.16) as well as clusters of small hemosiderin-laden particles, depicted as signal voids, in pigmented villonodular synovitis (Figs. 10.8, 10.9 and Figs. 17.32, 17.33).

Chronic Bursal Irritation

Chronic irritation of a bursa is primarily characterized by increased intrabursal fluid volumes, appearing as correspondingly larger areas of hyperintensity on relative or pure T2-weighting with signal reduction on T1-weighted images. Hemorrhagic components in the fluid may produce a slightly hyperintense signal on T1-weighting (Figs. 10.16–10.24).

10.6 Clinical Role of MRI Findings

MRI may contribute important information in differentiating fatty tissue proliferation of the infrapatellar fat pad (Hoffa's disease) from other conditions such as tumors.

A medial patellar plica of variable extent and shape is present in about half of all knees. Treatment

Table 10.1. Characteristic signal intensities

	T1w	T2w	T2*w	rho-w	FAT-SAT
Hoffa's fat pad	↑↑	↑	0	↑	0 – ↑
Fat pad tear	0 – ↑	↑↑ – ↑↑↑	↑↑ – ↑↑↑	↑↑	↑↑ – ↑↑↑
Fat pad inflammation	↑	↑ – ↑↑	↑ – ↑↑	↑↑	↑↑ – ↑↑↑
Bursitis	0 – ↑	↑↑↑	↑↑↑	↑↑	↑↑↑

0 No signal; ↑ low SI; ↑↑ intermediate SI; ↑↑↑ high SI.

is required only when this plica causes considerable clinical symptoms.

In demonstrating intra-articular loose bodies, conventional radiography and/or CT are superior to MRI in most cases.

Prepatellar bursitis is typically an ancillary finding at MRI. This condition can be diagnosed reliably in most cases without MRI. Nor does MRI contribute much to the differentiation of the various types of prepatellar bursitis, although it may be helpful in assessing its extent.

Further Reading

Boles CA, Ward WG SR (2000) Loose fragments and other debris: miscellaneous synovial and marrow disorders. Magn Reson Imaging Clin N Am 8 (2): 371–390

Jacobson JA, Lenchik L, Ruhoy MK, Schweitzer ME, Resnick D (1997) MR imaging of the infrapatellar fat pad of Hoffa. Radiographics 17 (3): 675–691

Jee WH, Choe BY, Kim JM, Song HH, Choi KH (1998) The plica syndrome: diagnostic value of MRI with arthroscopic correlation. J Comput Assist Tomogr 22 (5): 814–818

Nakanishi K, Inoue M, Ishida T, Murakami T, Tsuda K, Ikezoe J, Nakamura H (1996) MR evaluation of mediopatellar plica. Acta Radiol 37 (4): 567–571

Patel SJ, Kaplan PA, Dussault RG, Kahler DM (1998) Anatomy and clinical significance of the horizontal cleft in the infrapatellar fat pad of the knee: MR imaging. AJR Am J Roentgenol 170 (6): 1551–1555

Tang G, Niitsu M, Ikeda K, Endo H, Itai Y (2000) Fibrous scar in the infrapatellar fat pad after arthroscopy: MR imaging. Radiat Med 18 (1): 1–5

Fig. 10.1. Normal Hoffa's fat pad (18-year-old female)

Sagittal T1: Hyperintensity of Hoffa's fat pad isointense to sub-cutaneous fatty structures. Slight patella alta (Insall-Salvati ratio 1.32)

Fig. 10.2 a, b. Enlarged Hoffa's fat pad with pronounced posterior extension; discreet tears and impingement (19-year-old male)

a Sagittal T1: Pronounced posterior extension of Hoffa's fat pad with curvilinear central signal decreases

b Sagittal T2*: Extension of joint effusion into central cleft indicated by hyperintensity in an otherwise hypointense fat pad on relatively T2-weighted image

a

b

Fig. 10.3. Tear of Hoffa's fat pad (16-year-old male)

Sagittal; *left* T1, *right* T2*: Contour disruption of central fat pad depicted as curved band of reduced signal intensity on T1-weighted image and pronounced hyperintensity on relative T2-weighting. Slight joint effusion

Fig. 10.4. Extensive partial tears of superior Hoffa's fat pad, discreet inferior patellar fracture (12-year-old boy)

Sagittal; *left* T1, *right* T2*: Narrow zone of reduced signal intensity at inferior anterior margin of patella on T1-weighted image with increased signal intensity on relative T2-weighting (*arrows*) and contour disruption of inferior pole. In addition, wedge-shaped defects in superior aspect of fat pad with reduced signal intensity on T1-weighted image and increased signal intensity on relatively T2-weighted image. Slight joint effusion

Fig. 10.5 a, b. Extensive partial tear of Hoffa's fat pad; partial fatty tissue necrosis with calcification (47-year-old female)

a Sagittal T1; **b** sagittal T2*: Reduced signal intensity of posterosuperior aspect of Hoffa's fat pad with area of no signal at posterior margin on T1-weighted image (*arrow* in **a**); area of almost complete absence of signal also on relative T2-weighting (*arrow* in **b**). Slight joint effusion

a

b

**Fig. 10.6 a, b. Hoffa'itis
(46-year-old male)**

a Sagittal T1: Diffuse, partly netlike, signal decrease of almost entire fat pad on T1-weighted image due to extensive edema

b Sagittal T2*: Considerably increased signal intensity of central portion of fat pad on relatively T2-weighted image. Small contour defects of anterior and posterior margin. Slight joint effusion. Diffusely increased signal of prepatellar/infrapatellar subcutaneous structures, consistent with local reactive edema

Fig. 10.7 a, b. Synovial proliferation at posterior margin of Hoffa's fat pad; arthroscopy for chondromalacia patellae 2 years earlier (43-year-old female)

a Sagittal T1: Crescent area of decreased signal intensity in posterior two thirds of Hoffa's fat pad

b Sagittal T2*: Pronounced signal increase of this area on relatively T2-weighted image

a

b

a

b

c

d

Fig. 10.8 a–d. Suspected synovioma at posterior margin of Hoffa's fat pad – no surgery (56-year-old female)

a Coronal T1; **c** sagittal T1: Clearly defined ovoid tumor of homogeneously low signal intensity at posterior margin of Hoffa's fat pad

b Sagittal T2*: Central portions of the lesion showing slightly higher signal intensity compared to normal fat pad. Lesion surrounded by faint black margin. Isolated punctiform signal decreases suggesting focal pigmented villonodular synovitis as a differential diagnosis

d Contrast-enhanced sagittal T1: Moderate enhancement of the lesion

a

b

c

d

Fig. 10.9 a – d. Focal pigmented villonodular synovitis – histologically confirmed (67-year-old male)

a Coronal T1; **c** sagittal T1: Ovoid mass at posterior margin of Hoffa's fat pad similar as in Fig. 10.8, but with a small, satellite-like focus at the anterior margin of the anterior cruciate ligament attachment. In contrast to the preceding case, more inhomogeneous margins and decreased signal intensity, in particular in superior aspect (*arrow* in **c**)

b Sagittal T2*: Marked central hyperintensity of the lesion with posterior areas of lower intensity and absence of signal in superior aspect (*arrow*)

d Contrast-enhanced sagittal T1: Moderate contrast enhancement of the lesion except for superior/posterior marginal areas

a

b

c

d

Fig. 10.10 a – d. Ganglion cyst of Hoffa's fat pad (15-year-old male)

a Coronal T1; **c** sagittal T1: Both images show ovoid cystic lesion of decreased signal intensity at posterior margin of Hoffa's fat pad (*arrows*)

b Axial T2*; **d** sagittal T2*: Considerable hyperintensity of the lesion (in contrast to Figs. 10.8 and 10.9) with depiction of delicate septa (*arrows*)

a

b

c

d

Fig. 10.11 a – d. Large ganglion cyst of Hoffa's fat pad (27-year-old male)

a Sagittal T1; **c** coronal T1: Extensive lobulated cystic lesion in central/posterior Hoffa's fat pad with signal nearly isointense to muscle

b Sagittal T2*; **d** axial T2*: Considerable hyperintensity of lesion (as in Fig. 10.10) with depiction of multiple, delicate septations

Fig. 10.12. Slightly hypertrophic suprapatellar fat pad without irritation (29-year-old female)

Sagittal; *left* T1, *right* T2*: Normal fat signal of suprapatellar fat pad at the posterior margin of the quadriceps tendon insertion with slight posterior protrusion. Slight joint effusion (borderline)

Fig. 10.13. Edema of suprapatellar fat pad with partly detached portions (32-year-old male)

Sagittal; *left* T1, *right* T2*: Decreased signal intensity of suprapatellar fat pad compared to normal signal intensity of Hoffa's fat pad on T1-weighted image. Poorly defined. Relatively T2-weighted image (*right*) shows slight hyperintensity of suprapatellar fat pad compared to normal Hoffa signal with pronounced contour irregularities and cranial extension (*arrow*)

Fig. 10.14. Synovial proliferation or edema of suprapatellar fat pad with some mass effect (histology: chronic sclerosing synovitis; 45-year-old female)

Sagittal; *left* T1, *right* T2*: Well-defined, slightly hypertrophic suprapatellar fat pad with posterior convexity. Decreased signal intensity compared to normal signal of Hoffa's fat pad on T1-weighted image and increased signal on relative T2-weighting. Moderate joint effusion

Fig. 10.15. Intra-articular ganglion cyst in suprapatellar recess (40-year-old female)

Sagittal; *left* T1, *right* T2*: Lobulated cystic lesion in the area of the suprapatellar recess with soft tissue signal on T1-weighted image (*arrow*). In contrast to the lesions depicted in Figs. 10.13 and 10.14, this lesion shows marked hyperintensity on relative T2-weighting with just barely discernible septations (*arrow*)

Fig. 10.16a, b. Pronounced prepatellar bursitis (54-year-old female)

a Sagittal T1: Extensive crescent-shaped signal decrease of prepatellar bursa. Netlike signal decreases of adjacent subcutaneous structures

b Sagittal T2*: Extensive signal increase (equivalent to fluid) of prepatellar bursa with delicate extensions into infrapatellar subcutaneous structures

a

b

Fig. 10.17. Hematoma of pre-patellar bursa – contusion 2 weeks ago (47-year-old female)

Sagittal; *left* T1, *right* T2*: Compared to Fig. 10.16, T1-weighted image shows more pronounced hyperintensity, especially in superior aspect (*arrow*) of the massively enlarged, ovoid prepatellar bursa. Again with netlike signal decreases of directly adjacent structures and more diffuse signal decrease at the level of the deep infrapatellar bursa. Relatively T2-weighted image (*right*) depicting a circumscribed, markedly hyperintense fluid collection of the prepatellar bursa. Surrounding subcutaneous structures with diffusely increased signal intensity – again most prominent in infrapatellar area

Fig. 10.18. Chronic prepatellar bursitis following previous hematoma (59-year-old male)

Sagittal; *left* T1, *right* T2*: Reduced signal intensity of prepatellar bursa (equivalent to fluid) with partly netlike, suprapatellar and infra-patellar extensions on T1-weighted image. Moderately hyperintense signal on relatively T2-weighted image (*right*) with depiction of multiple small septa, suggesting a more long-standing process

Fig. 10.19. Chronic prepatellar bursitis with erosive defect of anterior patella (50-year-old male)

Sagittal; *left* T1, *right* T2*: Elongation and thickening of prepatellar bursa with reduced signal intensity on T1-weighted image and increased signal on relative T2-weighting. Bowl-shaped defect of anterior patella surrounded by black margin (*arrows*)

Fig. 10.20. Superficial infrapatellar bursitis; discreet tendinosis of inferior patellar tendon insertion (31-year-old male)

Sagittal; *left* T1, *right* T2*: Circumscribed signal decrease of the superficial infrapatellar bursa on T1-weighted image (*arrow*) with marked signal increase on relative T2-weighting. Slight corresponding signal changes also of distal insertion of patellar tendon. Only small fluid volume of prepatellar bursa (*arrowhead – right image*)

Fig. 10.21. Chronic superficial infrapatellar bursitis (39-year-old male)

Sagittal T1: Extensive signal decrease of superficial infrapatellar bursa on T1-weighted image with local contour thickening. Areas of slightly decreased signal intensity also in proximal subcutaneous structures

Fig. 10.22. Partially organized hematoma of superficial infrapatellar bursa – lower leg contusion 3 weeks earlier (35-year-old male)

Sagittal; *left* T1, *right* T2*: Extensive signal intensity decrease of the superficial infrapatellar bursa with slightly less pronounced signal decrease also of proximal subcutaneous structures on T1-weighted image – less pronounced hypointensity than in Fig. 10.21. Marked hyperintensity of the partly delineated superficial infrapatellar bursa on relatively T2-weighted image with some septation. Slightly inhomogeneous signal increase of proximal subcutaneous structures and discreet signal increases of patellar tendon

Fig. 10.23 a, b. Discreet chronic deep infrapatellar bursitis (32-year-old female)

a Sagittal T1: Decreased signal intensity of inferior portion of Hoffa's fat pad, most prominent near patellar tendon insertion

b Sagittal T2: Pronounced signal increase of this portion with slightly increased signal intensity of patellar tendon insertion

a

b

Fig. 10.24. Deep infrapatellar bursitis with debris (22-year-old male)

Sagittal; *left* T1, *right* T2*: T1-weighted image shows roughly triangular signal decrease of basal aspect of deep infrapatellar bursa with a slightly more hypointense central portion (*arrow*). Relatively T2-weighted image shows increased signal intensity (equivalent to fluid) with blurred delicate extensions into central part of Hoffa's fat pad. Slight signal increase also of distal patellar tendon insertion and mildly increased signal intensity of superficial infrapatellar bursa as slight concomitant reactions. Differential diagnosis: tendinosis with accompanying bursitis

11 Baker's Cysts, Ganglion Cysts

11.1 Technique and Method

T2-weighted MRI sequences are most suitable to locate cysts about the knee. Further characterization of such cysts in unusual locations or of unusual extent and configuration may require T1-weighted imaging before and after administration of an intravenous contrast medium.

11.2 Anatomy

The terms Baker's cyst and popliteal cyst are occasionally used to refer to all ganglion-like cystic lesions that occur in the popliteal area between the semimembranosus muscle and the medial head of the gastrocnemius muscle. Such popliteal cysts comprise the cystically transformed bursae of the semimembranosus and medial gastrocnemius muscles as well as Baker's cysts in the original sense of the term.

Baker's cysts as originally described by Baker (1877) by definition communicate directly with the knee joint via a stalk attached to the posterior joint capsule.

Ganglion cysts are fluid-filled benign tumors that typically arise in the soft tissue around tendon sheaths and joints but may also develop in cartilage (meniscal ganglion cysts) and para-articular bone (intraosseous ganglion cysts).

Histologically, the wall of ganglion cysts consists of connective tissue of variable cell content interspersed with edematous zones and areas of typical mucoid degeneration. Ganglion cysts contain a mucinous fluid with a high content of acid mucopolysaccarides.

11.3 Normal MRI Appearance

Small intra-articular zones with fluid signal (signal decrease on T1-weighting and increase on T2-weighting) represent normal findings, especially when they are located below the patella or in posterior areas of the joint, where they serve as reserve spaces, but not when they are extra-articular in location or contiguous with external capsular structures.

11.4 Pathomechanism

It is now widely held that popliteal cysts develop from herniations of the joint capsule or as retention cysts of the semimembranosus while meniscal ganglion cysts are assumed to arise on the basis of mucous degeneration of fibrous structures.

However, the etiology of ganglion cysts continues to be a controversial issue on which many different theories have been proposed, ranging from the assumption of traumatic degenerative causes to the view that ganglion cysts are true neoplastic tumors.

11.5 Pathophysiology

Popliteal cysts have a characteristic clinical presentation with circumscribed tender swelling in their typical location between the medial gastrocnemius muscle and the semimembranosus tendon – which has no direct relationship to the popliteal nerve and vessel bundle. The differentiation between true Baker's cysts (stalked) and ganglion cysts (unstalked) of the popliteal area continues to be important in terms of both therapy and prognosis.

A specific type of cyst is the so-called descended Baker's cyst, most likely due to rupture of the primary cyst with spilling of its content into the area of the lower leg, where it then becomes enclosed by a synovium-like membrane to form a secondary cyst. This type of Baker's cyst causes pronounced swelling in the area of the lower leg with extensive reactive local inflammation and, because of this clinical presentation, must be differentiated from deep vein thrombosis of the leg.

Meniscal ganglion cysts are much more common laterally than medially. This is because the lateral meniscus has a more voluminous anterior horn which can consequently develop a larger area of mucoid degeneration. Meniscal ganglion cysts arise as round to oval lateral outpouchings of such degenerated meniscal tissue and may occasionally communicate with the base of the meniscus by a stalk-like process.

Ganglion cysts of the lateral meniscus are frequently associated with meniscal damage (tear) while in the much rarer case of medial meniscal ganglion cysts the meniscus itself is typically intact.

11.6 MRI Signs of Abnormal Findings

Depending on their composition, intra- and extra-articular fluid collections may appear hyperintense (when they contain large amounts of protein, blood, or fat) or hypointense (serous effusion) on T1-weighted images. T2-weighted sequences typically depict all fluids as hyperintense.

Baker's cysts in the strict sense of the term may either contain pure fluid or fluid admixed with fat and blood components. Occasionally, they may be septated, contain debris, or have thrombotic areas.

The signal intensity of Baker's cysts varies with their contents: On T1-weighted images, debris may be of higher signal intensity or of lower signal intensity – especially when calcified – than the typical hypointense fluid signal. On T2-weighted images,

intracystic septa, loose bodies, and debris are delineated as marked hypointensities against the hyperintense fluid (Figs. 11.1 – 11.6).

Ganglion cysts have a more viscous content and are frequently septated. They are markedly hyperintense on T2-weighted images with the septa being delineated as hypointense structures. Ganglion cysts occur inside or outside the joint space. In both locations, they typically communicate with the joint capsule. This connection may be difficult to identify when it solely consists of a very discreet stalk-like process (Figs. 11.8 – 11.14).

Synovial plicae representing remnants of embryonic development, of which the three major types are suprapatellar, mediopatellar, and infrapatellar in location, can persist into adult life and are sometimes delineated as delicate linear hypointensities against the hyperintense joint fluid on T1-weighted images. Inflammation of such plicae is associated with thickening and surrounding exudative reactions.

11.7 Clinical Role of MRI Findings

Baker's cysts and (meniscal) ganglion cysts are excised surgically when they cause symptoms. In the case of meniscal ganglion cysts, preoperative arthroscopic assessment of the meniscus from which the cyst arises is required.

Popliteal cysts that do not communicate with the posterior joint capsule tend to recur less frequently than genuine Baker's cysts. When the latter are removed, care must be taken to radically excise the stalk. Moreover, it is advisable to search for and eliminate intra-articular causes of excess synovium production, the major cause of recurrent cysts.

Table 11.1. Characteristic signal intensities

	T1w	T2w	T2*w	rho-w	FAT-SAT
Effusion (serous)	0 – ↑	↑↑↑	↑↑↑	↑ – ↑↑	↑↑↑
Baker's cyst (simple)	0 – ↑	↑↑↑	↑↑ – ↑↑↑	↑ – ↑↑	↑↑↑
Baker's cyst (complicated)	↑ – ↑↑	↑↑ – ↑↑↑	↑↑ – ↑↑↑	↑↑	↑↑ – ↑↑↑

0 No signal; ↑ low SI; ↑↑ intermediate SI; ↑↑↑ high SI.

Further Reading

Baker NM (1877) Chronic disease of the knee joint – large cast in the cave. St. Barth Hosp Rep 13:254

Kulshrestha A, Misra RN, Agarwal P, Gupta D (1995) Magnetic resonance appearance of tuberculosis of the knee joint with ruptured Baker's cyst. Australas Radiol 39 (1): 80–83

Lang IM, Hughes DG, Williamson JB, Gough SG (1997) MRI appearance of popliteal cysts in childhood. Pediatr Radiol 27 (2): 130–132

Lektrakul N, Skaf A, Yeh L, Roger B, Schweitzer M, Blasbalg R, Resnick D (1999) Pericruciate meniscal cysts arising from tears of the posterior horn of the medial meniscus: MR imaging features that simulate posterior cruciate ganglion cysts. AJR Am J Roentgenol 172 (6): 1575–1579

Marti Bonmati L, Molla E, Dosda R, Casillas C, Ferrer P (2000) MR imaging of Baker cysts – prevalence and relation to internal derangements of the knee. MAGMA 10 (3): 205–210

Morrison JL, Kaplan PA (2000) Water on the knee: cysts, bursae, and recesses. Magn Reson Imaging Clin N Am 8 (2): 349–370

Munk PL, Vellet AD, Levin MF (1993) Leaking Baker's cyst detected by magnetic resonance imaging. Can Assoc Radiol J 44 (2): 125–128

Ohno Y, Itokazu M, Sakaeda H, Iinuma N, Shima H (1998) Meniscal cyst in the posterior intercondylar space found by magnetic resonance imaging. Arch Orthop Trauma Surg 117 (6–7): 394–396

Sansone V, de Ponti A, Paluello GM, del Maschio A (1995) Popliteal cysts and associated disorders of the knee. Critical review with MR imaging. Int Orthop 19 (5): 275–279

Sumen Y, Ochi M, Deie M, Adachi N, Ikuta Y (1999) Ganglion cysts of the cruciate ligaments detected by MRI. Int Orthop 23 (1): 58–60

Fig. 11.1 a, b. Baker's cyst (38-year-old female)

a Sagittal T2*; b axial T2*: Cystic lesion (*arrows*) between margin of medial gastrocnemius muscle and posterior margin of medial condyle with pronounced hyperintensity (equivalent to fluid) on relative T2*-weighting. Lesion partly lobulated and partly septated. In addition, delicate grade III tear of medial meniscal posterior horn

a

b

Fig. 11.2 a, b. Baker's cyst with debris/joint chondromas (60-year-old male)

a Sagittal T2*; **b** axial T2*: Typical cystic lesion at posterior margin of medial condyle with pronounced increase in signal intensity (equivalent to fluid) on relative T2-weighting containing isolated hypointense roundish loose bodies (*arrows*)

a

b

c

Fig. 11.3 a–c. Baker's cyst with partly ossified joint chondromas; tear of medial meniscus; gonarthosis (78-year-old male)

a Sagittal T1: Ovoid cystic lesion at posterior margin of medial condyle of low signal intensity on T1-weighted image containing circular loose bodies of either absent or marrow signal intensity (*arrow*). Posterior horn of medial meniscus no longer fully delineated. Absent signal intensity indicates definite sclerosis of tibial articular surface with a more pronounced subchondral reaction

b Sagittal T2*; **c** axial T2*: Baker's cyst with increased signal intensity (equivalent to fluid) containing isolated hypointense roundish loose bodies. Extensive defects of posterior horn of medial meniscus. Tibia showing slightly increased subchondral signal intensity with massive thinning of articular cartilage

**Fig. 11.4a, b. Large Baker's cyst
(53-year-old male)**

a Sagittal T1; **b** sagittal T2*: Ovoid
cystic lesion isointense to fluid at
medial margin of gastrocnemius
muscle; markedly hypointense
on T1-weighted image and hyperintense on relative T2-weighting

**Fig. 11.5. Large Baker's cyst with
involvement of pes anserinus bursa
(57-year-old female)**

Axial T2*: Baker's cyst in typical
location between posterior margin
of medial condyle and medial
gastrocnemius muscle but with
additional anteromedial extension
toward pes anserinus. Pronounced
signal increase on relative
T2-weighting

Fig. 11.6 a, b. Baker's cyst with involvement of pes anserinus bursa (65-year-old female)

a Sagittal T2*; **b** axial T2*: Markedly hyperintense fluid collection at posteromedial proximal tibial plateau in the vicinity of the sartorius tendon. Central degeneration of posterior horn of medial meniscus, grade II

a

b

Fig. 11.7 a, b. Chronic irritation of pes anserinus bursa (59-year-old female)

a Sagittal T2*; **b** axial T2*: Delicate, slightly convex area of increased signal intensity (equivalent to fluid) in the vicinity of the distal sartorius tendon/medial tibial plateau insertion site of pes anserinus (*arrows*)

Fig. 11.8 a, b. Large ganglion cyst at tibiofibular joint with inferior extension (25-year-old male)

a Sagittal T2; b coronal T2: Very large, lobulated cystic lesion in retrotibial/paratibial area, directly anterior to the proximal tibio-fibular joint. T2-weighted images show very pronounced increase in signal intensity and multiple intralesional septa

a

b

c

d

Fig. 11.9a–d. Lateral capsular ganglion cyst with superior extension (38-year-old female)

a Coronal T1; **c** sagittal T1: Lobulated cystic lesion of grapelike appearance at superior margin of lateral condyle lateral to distal femoral metaphysis. Signal nearly isointense to muscle

b Axial T2*; **d** sagittal T2*: Pronounced signal increase of the lesion. Delicate septations much more conspicuous than on T1-weighting

a

b

Fig. 11.10 a, b. **Posterior capsular ganglion cyst with intra-articular extension (43-year-old female)**

a Sagittal T2*; **b** axial T2*: Lobulated cystic lesion in the area of the posterior capsule with intra-articular portions at posterior margin of posterior cruciate ligament. Relatively T2-weighted images show marked hyperintensity of the lesion and isolated septations (*arrows*)

Fig. 11.11 a, b. Posterior (lateral) capsular ganglion cyst without intra-articular extension (33-year-old male)

a Sagittal T2*; **b** axial T2*: Extra-articular, lobulated, partly septated cystic lesion in para-median location at posterior cap-sular margin with markedly in-creased signal intensity on relative T2-weighting (*arrows*)

Fig. 11.12a, b. Very large postero-lateral capsular ganglion cyst (27-year-old male)

a Sagittal T2*; **b** axial T2*: Extensive lobulated, partly septated cystic lesion at posterior margin of lateral condyle communicating with superior capsular attachment. Pronounced signal increase on relative T2-weighting

a

b

Fig. 11.13a, b. Large medial meniscal ganglion cyst (39-year-old male)

a Coronal T2; **b** axial T2*: Both images show ovoid, partly septated fluid collection of markedly increased signal intensity contiguous with medial joint cleft areas. Connection to medial meniscus not seen but likely since there is central meniscal degeneration (*not shown*)

a

b

Fig. 11.14a, b. Lateral meniscal ganglion cyst and peripheral tear (40-year-old female)

a Coronal T2*: Ovoid fluid collection at peripheral margin of lateral meniscus adjacent to wedge-shaped contour defect of meniscus (*arrow*)

b Axial T2: Purely T2-weighted image likewise shows marked hyperintensity of the lesion at lateral joint cleft. Only faintly seen septa

a

b

Fig. 11.15 a, b. Ossified capsular/ articular chondroma in posterior recess (35-year-old female)

a Sagittal T1; **b** sagittal T2*: Ovoid formation in posterior capsular recess contiguous with capsule. Both sequences show lesion with decreased signal intensity and some central areas of increased signal intensity. Slight reactive effusion

a

b

Fig. 11.16a, b. Ossified capsular/ articular chondroma, located medially in posterosuperior recess (42-year-old male)

a Sagittal T1; **b** sagittal T2*: Roundish element of marrow signal in posterosuperior joint recess at proximal posterior margin of medial condyle. Moderate joint effusion. Empty medial meniscal posterior recess following meniscectomy 4 years earlier. Chondral damage in medial compartment

a

b

Fig. 11.17 a, b. Small fabella posterior to lateral condyle (75-year-old female)

a Sagittal T1; **b** sagittal T2*: Small extra bony structure resembling a sesamoid situated outside the joint space at posterior margin of posterior capsule of lateral condyle (*arrows*)

a

b

Fig. 11.18. Posteromedial capsular calcification – repeat trauma (33-year-old male)

Sagittal; *left* T1, *right* T1: Slightly thickened contour of posterior capsule of conspicuously low to absent signal intensity (*arrows*)

12 Popliteal Vessels

12.1 Technique and Method

The vessels can be best imaged in sagittal and axial orientations. MR angiography may yield useful additional information in specific cases.

12.2 Anatomy

The popliteal artery runs straight between the heads of the gastrocnemius muscle. When there is complete interruption of flow in this artery, collateral circulation cannot be maintained by the geniculate arteries. On the venous side, there are often several parallel popliteal veins.

12.3 Normal MRI Appearance

Normal vessels typically appear very hypointense on T1-weighted images, hyperintense on relatively T2-weighted images, and hypointense on purely T2-weighted images.

Reduction of flow velocity results in increasing signal intensity on T1-weighted images and may possibly be associated with a decrease in signal intensity on relatively T2-weighted images. However, flow-related signal changes are inconsistent and must be interpreted with caution.

12.4 Pathomechanism

Most arterial injuries are caused by dislocation of the knee joint, which may have undergone spontaneous repositioning at the time of examination. This must be borne in mind in all patients presenting with severe knee injury and warrants evaluation of arterial flow.

Moreover, vessels may be damaged inadvertently in knee surgery such as posterior cruciate ligament reconstruction, in which unnoticed marginal or complete lesions of the popliteal vessels may occur, and meniscectomy with excision of large parts of the posterior horns. The latter is primarily associated with the development of false popliteal aneurysms.

False popliteal aneurysms also occur in sutured vessels, in particular in the area of suture of prosthetic implants. True aneurysms typically develop on the basis of atherosclerotic vessel damage. Venous injuries pose a problem because they may be associated with local thrombus formation.

12.5 Pathophysiology

Arterial injuries in the popliteal region with interruption of arterial flow frequently cause ischemia in the area of the calf and foot (compartmental syndromes), which may require amputation. Collateral circulation is rarely adequate.

Venous thrombi of the popliteal region can be collateralized by accompanying veins and the superficial veins of the knee. Clinically significant are floating thrombi of the popliteal area because they may cause pulmonary embolism.

12.6 MRI Signs of Abnormal Findings

In addition to the identification of abnormal flow signals, MRI is performed to assess the vessel wall for fusiform or sacculated dilatations/aneurysms and varicosis as well as for the presence of calcification (indicated by black margins).

Thickening of the vessel wall isointense to soft tissue is primarily caused by thrombotic material. A streaky appearance of a vessel may suggest central thrombi.

12.7 Clinical Role of MRI Findings

Any obstruction of arterial or venous flow in the major vessels of the knee area represents a serious disorder requiring appropriate treatment. Arterial obstruction in most cases requires interventions to reestablish patency while obstruction of venous drainage can be treated conservatively.

Mistaking an arterial aneurysm with displacement of venous drainage and peripheral edema formation for early thrombosis may have serious consequences.

Further Reading

Atilla S, Akpek ET, Yucel C, Tali ET, Isik S (1998) MR imaging and MR angiography in popliteal artery entrapment syndrome. Eur Radiol 8 (6): 1025–1029

Pomeranz SJ (1991) Orthopaedic MRI. JB Lippincott, Philadelphia

Smith PN, Gelinas J, Kennedy K, Thain L, Rorabeck CH, Bourne RB (1999) Popliteal vessels in knee surgery. A magnetic resonance imaging study. Clin Orthop (367): 158–164

Table 12.1. Characteristic signal intensities

	T1w	T2w	T2*w	rho-w	FAT-SAT
Blood vessels	0 – ↑	0 – ↑↑	↑↑ – ↑↑↑	↑	↑
Thrombus	↑ – ↑↑	↑↑	↑	↑	↑ – ↑↑

0 No signal; ↑ low SI; ↑↑ intermediate SI; ↑↑↑ high SI.

a

b

c

d

Fig. 12.1a–d. Popliteal aneurysm with partial thrombosis (67-year-old male)

a Sagittal T1: Fusiform to saccular dilatation of the popliteal artery at the level of the femoral condyles. Signal intensity nearly isointense to soft tissue with a tubular center of lower intensity (*arrow*) and delicate black margins (*arrowhead*)

b Coronal T1: Area of intraluminal flow clearly delineated as a low-signal-intensity bandlike structure against the slightly more hyperintense thrombotic marginal areas

c Sagittal – intermediately weighted 3D acquisition: Hyperintensity of areas of flow in the popliteal artery (*arrow*) and lower intensity of thrombotic areas (*arrowhead*)

d Sagittal – 3D reconstruction from intermediately weighted sequence: Course of intraluminal flow clearly depicted as hyperintensity while thrombotic material is only very poorly differentiated

Fig. 12.2. Posttraumatic giant aneurysm of popliteal artery with partial thrombosis – knee distortion 3 weeks earlier (56-year-old male)

Sagittal T2*: Huge popliteal aneurysm with hyperintense anterior portions indicating flow and lamellar marginal layers of slightly less pronounced hyperintensity. Black marginal areas consistent with thrombotic material and calcification

a

b

c

d

Fig. 12.3a–d. Chronic popliteal aneurysm, thrombotic and partly calcified; status post popliteal reconstruction/bypass (45-year-old male)

a Sagittal T1; **b** coronal T1: Hyperintense popliteal aneurysm surrounded by black margins. Central hyperintensity due to clotted blood components. Coronal section depicts part of the vessel bypass as a thread-like structure medial to the aneurysm (*arrow*)

c, d Sagittal T2*: Depiction of markedly hyperintense circular lesion surrounded by a black margin with slight irregularities toward the center – bypass segment depicted anteromedially as a hyperintense band with a screw-like appearance (*arrow* in **d**)

a

b

c

d

Fig. 12.4a–d. Chronic popliteal vein thrombosis (59-year-old male)

a, b Sagittal T1: Conspicuously hyperintense popliteal vein (*arrows*) posterior to the very hypointense artery

c Sagittal T2*; **d** axial T2*: Slightly hypointense, somewhat heterogeneous signal of the popliteal vein with prominent marginal area of lower signal intensity (*arrows*)

13 Retropatellar Degeneration (Chondromalacia, Osteochondritis Dissecans)

13.1 Technique and Method

The articular cartilage of the patella can best be assessed on T2*-weighted and fat-suppressed images acquired in axial and sagittal orientations.

13.2 Anatomy

Degenerative changes of the articular cartilage (softening) of the patella affect both the medial and the lateral articular surface.

Osteochondritis dissecans of the patella may likewise involve the lateral and/or medial facet and frequently occurs bilaterally (in up to 30% of cases). The majority of osteochondral lesions are found in the distal third of the patella.

13.3 Normal MRI Appearance

The retropatellar cartilage is the thickest articular cartilage of the human locomotor system, measuring 5–10 mm in its central portion. The cartilage is of intermediate signal intensity on T1-weighted and T2-weighted images and is smoothly marginated both toward the subchondral bone and the joint space. Central areas of slightly decreased signal intensity represent normal variation (Fig. 13.3).

13.4 Pathomechanism

Chondromalacia patellae is a degenerative disorder of cartilage caused by an imbalance of loading and loading capacity of the articular cartilage, resulting either from excessive loading (congenital or acquired deformities or overuse associated with certain occupations or sporting activities) or from a reduced loading capacity (idiopathic arthropathy).

Osteochondritis dissecans is a circumscribed bone necrosis in which the overlying articular cartilage is initially intact.

13.5 Pathophysiology

Both chondromalacia patellae and osteochondritis dissecans are graded in terms of clinical and therapeutic factors.

Grading of chondromalacia patellae (e.g. according to Outerbridge):

Grade I: Softening of the cartilage with loss of staining.
Grade II: Superficial fragmentation and fissuring.
Grade III: Defects extending to the underlying bone (up to 2 cm).
Grade IV: Exposure of the subchondral bone with sclerotic changes (extensive).

In osteochondritis dissecans, the following clinical/arthroscopic stages are distinguished:

1. Initial stage (characterized by acute necrosis and initial structural loosening).
2. Sclerotic stage (intact articular cartilage).
3. Fragmentation stage (elastic cartilage).
4. Final stage (complete healing or incomplete healing with persistence of a partly or completely detached osteochondral fragment).

13.6 MRI Signs of Abnormal Findings

Bipartite Patella

Demonstration of one or more isolated bone fragments, typically located in the superolateral aspect of the patella (male-female ratio 9 to 1). Unilateral in 50% of cases. Cleft filled with fibrous tissue or cartilage of typical signal intensity but not with fluid. Intact articular cartilage including portion overlying the cleft (Figs. 13.1 and 13.2).

Chondromalacia Patellae

The most widely used MRI grading system of chondromalacia patellae distinguishes *4 grades* of osteochondral damage that correlate with the clinical stages of the disease (see above – Sect. 13.5):

Grade I: Intrachondral edema as a substrate of cartilage softening, may be depicted as hypointensity. Only minor contour thickening – changes typically not seen at arthroscopy (Figs. 13.4–13.6).

Grade II: More pronounced contour thickening and irregularities as well as intrachondral signal decreases – changes detectable by arthroscopy (Figs. 13.7–13.9).

Grade III: Deep cartilage defects that may extend to the underlying bone, "crab meat" appearance of the surface (Figs. 13.10–13.12).

Grade IV: Deep cartilage ulceration extending to the underlying bone with subchondral reaction/initial detritus cyst formation: pronounced decreases in subchondral signal intensity on T1-weighted images and increased signal on relative T2-weighting (Figs. 13.13–13.16).

However, extremely exact grading of chondromalacia is less important than the identification of flaps and intra-articular loose bodies (when these are suspected on MRI, supplementary conventional radiography is mandatory).

Posttraumatic Injuries

- Transchondral damage.
- Osteochondral damage.
- Osteochondritis dissecans (may in principle also occur on the basis of degenerative changes associated with detritus cyst formation).

MRI Grading of Osteochondritis Dissecans

MRI grading closely correlates with the clinical/arthroscopic stages (see above – Sect. 13.5):

Grade I: Intact articular cartilage (lesion confined to bone).

Grade II: Partly delineated osteochondral fragment (Fig. 13.18).

Grade III: Fully delineated or detached osteochondral fragment – unstable finding (Fig. 13.19).

Grade IV: Detached and displaced osteochondral fragment (Fig. 13.20).

13.7 Clinical Role of MRI Findings

In patients with proven chondromalacia patellae, the underlying cause should be determined. Causative therapy for a reduced loading capacity of the articular cartilage (idiopathic chondromalacia) continues to be lacking.

When chondromalacia is due to excessive loading, the aim of therapy should be to reduce loading, e.g. by surgical correction.

Treatment of osteochondritis dissecans depends on the patient's age and the stage of the disease.

Conservative treatment is preferred in children until about age 10, as there is a high incidence of spontaneous regression in early childhood. Older patients in whom the overlying cartilage is intact may be treated by antegrade drilling of the necrotic lesion for interruption of the sclerotic zone.

Patients with a large necrotic focus or instability (elastic articular cartilage) frequently benefit from bony patching of the defect underlying intact articular cartilage. A completely or partly detached fragment may be removed surgically or reattached when both the detached cartilage and the underlying bone are still vital.

Regarding the role of MRI, it must be noted that it is limited in that it only allows for assessing the vitality of the marrow space tissue but provides no direct information on the vitality of the bone.

Intra-articular loose bodies frequently escape detection by MRI; assessment of (prior) supplementary conventional radiographs is recommended.

Further Reading

Aglietti P, Insall JN, Buzzi R et al. (1983) Idiopathic osteonecrosis of the knee: etiology, prognosis and treatment. J Bone Joint Surg 65B: 588–597

Ahn JM, Kwak SM, Kang HS et al. (1998) Evaluation of patellar cartilage in cadavers with a low-field-strength extremity-only magnetic comparison of MR imaging sequences with macroscopic findings as the standard. Radiology 208 (1): 57–62

Andresen R, Radmer S, Konig H, Banzer D, Wolf KJ (1996) MR diagnosis of retropatellar chondral lesions under compression. A comparison with histological findings. Acta Radiol 37 (1): 91–97

Burkart A, Imhoff AB (2000) Bildgebung nach autologer Chondrozytentransplantation. Korrelation kernspintomographischer, histologischer und arthroskopischer Befunde. SO: Orthopäde 29 (2): 135–144

Carrillon Y, Abidi H, Dejour D, Fantino O, Moyen B, Tran Minh VA (2000) Patellar instability: assessment on MR images by measuring the lateral trochlear inclination-initial experience. Radiology 216 (2): 582–585

Daenen BR, Ferrara MA, Marcelis S, Dondelinger RF (1998) Evaluation of patellar cartilage surface lesions: comparison of CT arthrography and fat-suppressed FLASH 3D MR imaging. Eur Radiol 8 (6): 981–985

Drape JL, Pessis E, Auleley GR, Chevrot A, Dougados M, Ayral X (1998) Quantitative MR imaging evaluation of chondropathy in osteoarthritic knees. Radiology 208 (1): 49–55

Hayes CW (1994) MRI of the patellofemoral joint. Semin Ultrasound CT MR 15 (5): 383–395

Leersum van M, Schweitzer ME, Gannon F, Finkel G, Vinitski S, Mitchell DG (1996) Chondromalacia patellae: an in vitro study. Comparison of MR criteria with histologic and macroscopic findings. Skeletal Radiol 25 (8): 727–732

Muellner T, Funovics M, Nikolic A, Metz V, Schabus R, Vecsei V (1998) Patellar alignment evaluated by MRI. Acta Orthop Scand 69 (5): 489–492

Muhle C, Brinkmann G, Skaf A, Heller M, Resnick D (1999) Effect of a patellar realignment brace on patients with patellar subluxation and dislocation. Evaluation with kinematic magnetic resonance imaging. Am J Sports Med 27 (3): 350–353

Outerbridge RE (1964) The etiology of chondromalacia patellae. J Bone Joint Surg 46B: 179

Rand T, Brossmann J, Pedowitz R, Ahn JM, Haghigi P, Resnick D (2000) Analysis of patellar cartilage. Comparison of conventional MR imaging and MR and CT arthrography in cadavers. Acta Radiol 41 (5): 492– 497

Sittek H, Eckstein F, Gavazzeni A, Milz S, Kiefer B, Schulte E, Reiser M (1996) Assessment of normal patellar cartilage volume and thickness using MRI: an analysis of currently available pulse sequences. Skeletal Radiol 25 (1): 55–62

Stäubli HU, Durrenmatt U, Porcellini B, Rauschning W (1999) Anatomy and surface geometry of the patellofemoral joint in the axial plane. J Bone Joint Surg Br 81 (3): 452–458

Wang SF, Cheng HC, Chang CY (1999) Fat-suppressed three-dimensional fast spoiled gradient-recalled echo imaging: a modified FS 3D SPGR technique for assessment of patellofemoral joint chondromalacia. Clin Imaging 23 (3): 177–180

Table 13.1. Characteristic signal intensities

	T1w	T2w	T2*w	rho-w	FAT-SAT
Cartilage	↑ – ↑↑	↑ – ↑↑	↑↑ – ↑↑↑	↑↑	↑↑ – ↑↑↑
Cartilage edema	↑↑	↑↑ – ↑↑↑	↑↑↑	↑↑	↑↑ – ↑↑↑
Mucoid degeneration	0 – ↑	↑↑ – ↑↑↑	↑↑↑	↑	↑↑ – ↑↑↑
Cartilage degeneration with loss of texture	0 – ↑	↑ – ↑↑	↑↑	0 – ↑	↑ – ↑↑
Osteochondritis dissecans	0 – ↑	↑ – ↑↑	↑ – ↑↑	↑	↑↑

0 No signal; ↑ low SI; ↑↑ intermediate SI; ↑↑↑ high SI.

Fig. 13.1 a, b. Lateral bipartite patella (45-year-old male)

a Coronal T1: Isolated lateral patellar fragment, cleft surrounded by absent signal intensity (*arrow*)

b Axial T2*: Vertical cleft through lateral patella of slightly hyperintense signal intensity (*arrow*). Articular cartilage intact including portion overlying the cleft

a

b

Fig. 13.2 a–d. Superolateral bipartite patella (55-year-old male)

a Coronal T1: Isolated superolateral patellar fragment, cleft surrounded by absent signal intensity (*arrow*)

b Sagittal T2*: Isolated superior patellar fragment delineated by a delicate band of slightly higher signal intensity (*arrow*). Intact articular cartilage. Slight joint effusion

c, d Axial T2*: Isolated patellar fragment separated by a slightly hyperintense cleft – intact articular cartilage

Fig. 13.3. Normal retropatellar articular cartilage (31-year-old male)

Axial T2*: Entirely homogeneous articular cartilage without thickening or signal changes

Fig. 13.4. Chondromalacia patellae, grade I (31-year-old male)

Axial T2*: Marked thickening of articular cartilage centrally (*arrow*)

Fig. 13.5. Chondromalacia patellae, grade I (to II) – (23-year-old female)

Axial T2*: Slight contour thickening of articular cartilage on the medial facet (*arrow*) with discreet structural loosening and barely visible irregularities more distally

Fig. 13.6. Chondromalacia patellae, grade I – II (16-year-old female)

Axial T2*: Rather flat patella with thickening of articular cartilage in central area. Circumscribed prominent area of reduced signal intensity over the medial facet with slight surface irregularity distally

Fig. 13.7. Chondromalacia patellae, grade II/chondral fracture following distortion, hunter's cap patella (21-year-old female)

Axial T2*: Pronounced thickening and signal decrease of articular cartilage on the lateral facet. Some sharply edged contour disruption with slight step formation

Fig. 13.8. Chondromalacia patellae, grade II (26-year-old male)

Axial T2*: Partial thinning of articular cartilage with surface irregularities over the lateral facet and centrally (*arrow*)

Fig. 13.9 a, b. Chondromalacia patellae, grade II (to III) following recurrent patellar dislocation in patellofemoral dysplasia (25-year-old male)

a, b Axial T2*: Considerable irregularities of articular cartilage centrally and at beginning of medial facet with deep contour defects, in part almost reaching underlying bone

a

b

Fig. 13.10. Chondromalacia patellae, grade II – III, hunter's cap patella (29-year-old male)

Axial T2*: Central defect of articular cartilage on the lateral facet (hunter's cap) with contour thickening, slight irregularities, and signal decreases of adjacent cartilage

Fig. 13.11. Chondromalacia patellae, grade II – III (39-year-old female)

Axial T2*: Articular cartilage markedly thinned medially with exposure of subchondral bone at the beginning of the medial facet (*arrow*). Slight reactive effusion. Small subcutaneous parapatellar fluid collection laterally

Fig. 13.12. Chondromalacia patellae, grade III, medial facet (58-year-old male)

Axial T2*: Exposure of underlying bone centrally/beginning of medial facet – somewhat prominent bony edges of peripheral patellar margins. Joint effusion

Fig. 13.13. Chondromalacia patellae, grade IV, reactive effusion (55-year-old female)

Axial T2*: Extensive exposure of underlying bone centrally and laterally. Small subchondral foci of increased signal intensity. Irregularities of articular cartilage on lateral femoral articular surface. Pronounced reactive effusion

Fig. 13.14. Retropatellar arthrosis/ chondromalacia patellae, grade IV (55-year-old female)

Sagittal T1: Prominent bony edges of posterior patellar poles. Pronounced sclerosis of posterior surface indicated by absent signal intensity. Pronounced subchondral signal decreases centrally (*arrow*). Slight joint effusion

Fig. 13.15. Retopatellar arthrosis/chondromalacia patellae, grade IV (55-year-old female)

Sagittal T2*: Prominent edges of posterior patellar poles. Exposure of underlying bone centrally with pronounced subchondral signal increase in this area (*arrow*). Slight joint effusion

Fig. 13.16 a, b. Chondromalacia patellae, grade II (to IV in inferior aspect), intrapatellar osteonecrotic zone/emerging detritus cyst (38-year-old male)

a Sagittal T2*; **b** axial T2*: Ovoid subchronal area of increased signal intensity in inferolateral patella with black margin. Overlying articular cartilage markedly thinned, partly with exposure of underlying bone (*arrow* in **a**)

a

b

Fig. 13.17a, b. Patellar detritus cyst/osteonecrosis/transition to osteochondritis dissecans – local chondromalacia, grade II (40-year-old male)

a Sagittal T2*; **b** axial T2*: Ovoid central defect of patella with pronounced increase in signal intensity on relatively T2-weighted images. Only small, incomplete cortical bridge. Thickening, loosening, and slight irregularity of articular cartilage

Fig. 13.18. Retropatellar osteochondritis dissecans, grade II (15-year-old male)

Axial T2*: Rather flat patella with nearly semicircular medial increase in signal intensity containing a nearly completely delineated area of lower intensity laterally (*arrow*). Overlying articular cartilage intact but slightly thickened

Fig. 13.19. Retropatellar osteo-chondritis dissecans, grade II – III (13-year-old girl)

Axial T2*: Lateral bowl-shaped contour defect of posterior surface of patella with a nearly completely isolated, mildly hypointense area. Thinning of overlying articular cartilage at the margins of this defect (*arrowheads*). Wiberg type III patellar variant tending toward hunter's cap. Slight reactive effusion

Fig. 13.20. Chronic retropatellar osteochondritis dissecans, grade IV (15-year-old male)

Axial T2*: Irregular central defect of posterior patellar surface. Local defect of overlying articular cartilage with elevation of a flap-like part medially (*arrow*). Considerable reactive effusion

14 Femorotibial Degeneration (Chondromalacia, Osteochondritis Dissecans, Spontaneous Osteonecrosis)

14.1 Technique and Method

Imaging in coronal and sagittal planes is most suitable and may be supplemented by axial sections, especially in assessing osteochondritis. Fat-suppressed sequences are likewise helpful. Intravenous contrast medium administration may help to assess the vitality of detached fragments but is usually not necessary when taking into account the signal characteristics.

14.2 Anatomy

Degenerative conditions may affect *both* (lateral and medial) compartments of the knee joint and frequently also involve the femoropatellar joint. Specific manifestations in *one* compartment (after trauma or in individuals with deformities such as genu varum or valgum) are more common medially than laterally.

Osteochondritis dissecans of the knee almost exclusively involves the medial femoral condyle at the transition to the intercondylar fossa.

In contrast, spontaneous osteonecrosis (Ahlbäck's disease) affects the loading zone of the medial femoral condyle.

14.3 Normal MRI Appearance

The hyaline articular cartilage of the patella, femur, and tibia is depicted as a homogeneous band of intermediate signal intensity that is smoothly marginated both toward the joint surface and toward the underlying cortical bone.

Precise assessment of the femorotibial articular cartilage by MRI is more difficult than of the patellar cartilage unless 3D acquisition with thin-slice reconstruction is used.

14.4 Pathomechanism

Degenerative damage of the femorotibial joint results from an imbalance between loading and loading capacity (see chondromalacia patellae).

Osteochondritis dissecans is a circumscribed aseptic necrosis involving a more or less extensive area of subchondral bone.

Osteonecrosis of the medial femoral condyle (Ahlbäck's disease) is a disease affecting older individuals (Figs. 14.11–14.14). A primary (idiopathic) form is distinguished from secondary osteonecrosis typically occurring after local corticosteroid treatment.

14.5 Pathophysiology

Four stages of femorotibial arthritis (arthritis of the knee joint) are distinguished on the basis of clinical and radiologic criteria.

Osteochondritis dissecans of the knee occurs bilaterally in up to 50% of patients. Staging is the same as for osteochondritis of other locations (developmental stages I–IV, cf. Sect. 13.5).

Osteonecrosis of the femoral condyle (Ahlbäck's disease) is classified into 5 radiologic grades (according to Aglietti et al. 1983):

Grade I: Normal radiograph.
Grade II: Flattening of the medial femoral condyle.
Grade III: Osteolysis with marginal sclerosis.
Grade IV: Collapse of subchondral bone resulting in a dense calcified plate.
Grade V: Secondary arthritis.

14.6 MRI Signs of Abnormal Findings

Femorotibial Chondromalacia

The MRI grading of femorotibial chondromalacia corresponds to that of chondromalacia patellae and distinguishes the following *grades*:

Grade I: Intrachondral edema with slight local decreases in signal intensity, no surface changes; normal arthroscopy (Fig. 14.6).

Grade II: Slight irregularities of articular cartilage, contour thickening and pronounced signal decreases; changes detectable by arthroscopy (Fig. 14.7).

Grade III: Deep cartilage defects that may extend to the underlying bone but without osseous reaction, in part "crab meat" appearance of the surface (Fig. 14.8).

Grade IV: Deep cartilage defects extending to the underlying bone with reactive bone changes/beginning detritus cyst formation: decreased signal intensity on T1-weighted images and increased signal intensity on T2*-weighting (Figs. 14.9 and 14.10).

As in chondromalacia patellae, it is again more important to identify detached chondral flaps and intra-articular loose bodies than to achieve a precise grading in all segments.

Correlation with radiographic findings is required in all cases where the MRI findings suggest a loose body.

Osteochondritis Dissecans

MRI grading taking into account the temporal course and severity of the disorder is as follows:

Grade I: Intact articular cartilage (lesion confined to bone): Subchondral decrease in signal intensity on T1-weighted image and increase on relatively T2-weighted image, especially in the area of femoral pressure-bearing zones (Figs. 14.1 and 14.2).

Grade II: Partly delineated osteochondral fragment: Area of reduced signal intensity on T1-weighted image separated by slight margin (black). Hyperintense edematous zones on T2-weighted image likewise delineated by partly black margins. Lamellar hyperintensities in this area due to synovial fluid extending into the cleft between the intact bone and the fragment (Figs. 14.3 and 14.4).

Grade III: Fully delineated or detached osteochondral fragment: Complete delineation of the fragment from the underlying bone by a black margin. Hyperintense cleft on relative T2-weighting; unstable finding (Fig. 14.5).

Grade IV: Detached and displaced osteochondral fragment: Wide distance between the detached fragment and the native bone or empty mouse bed.

14.7 MRI Pitfalls in Osteochondritis Dissecans

Osteochondritis dissecans must not be confused with slight developmental irregularities of (mostly posterior) condylar epiphyseal surfaces.

14.8 Clinical Role of MRI Findings

In all cases of femorotibial cartilage degeneration, an attempt should be made to determine the etiology, in particular when there is manifestation at an atypical age.

There is a steady increase with age of degenerative joint damage, especially of the highly loaded joints (hip and knee). All individuals over 60 will show degenerative cartilage changes of the knee when proper detection methods are used.

Arthropathy due to a reduced loading capacity of the articular cartilage currently lacks causative therapy. When arthropathy is due to excessive loading, the preferred treatment is to reduce loading. This may require surgery, especially in patients with deformities (genu varum/genu valgum and others).

The treatment of osteochondritis dissecans primarily depends on the patient's age and the stage of the disease. MRI in combination with conventional radiography yields important information, especially for surgery planning.

Table 14.1. Characteristic signal intensities

	T1w	T2w	T2*w	rho-w	FAT-SAT
Cartilage	↑ – ↑↑	↑ – ↑↑	↑↑ – ↑↑↑	↑↑	↑↑ – ↑↑↑
Cartilage edema	↑↑	↑↑ – ↑↑↑	↑↑↑	↑↑	↑↑ – ↑↑↑
Mucoid degeneration	0 – ↑	↑↑ – ↑↑↑	↑↑↑	↑	↑↑ – ↑↑↑
Cartilage degeneration with loss of texture	0 – ↑	↑ – ↑↑	↑↑	0 – ↑	↑ – ↑↑
Osteochondritis dissecans	0 – ↑	↑ – ↑↑	↑ – ↑↑	↑	↑↑

0 No signal; ↑ low SI; ↑↑ intermediate SI; ↑↑↑ high SI.

Further Reading

Aglietti P, Insall JN, Buzzi R et al. (1983) Idiopathic osteonecrosis of the knee: etiology, prognosis and treatment. J Bone Joint Surg 65B: 588–597

Bachmann G, Jurgensen I, Rominger M, Rau WS (1999) Die Bedeutung der Magnetresonanztomographie für die Verlaufskontrolle der Osteochondrosis dissecans am Knie- und Sprunggelenk. Rofo Fortschr Geb Röntgenstr Neuen Bildgeb Verfahr 171 (5): 372–379

Bachmann G, Jurgensen I, Siaplaouras J (1995) Die Studienbestimmung der Osteochondrosis dissecans am Knie- und Sprunggelenk mit der MRT. Vergleich mit konventioneller Radiologie und Arthroskopie. Rofo Fortschr Geb Röntgenstr Neuen Bildgeb Verfahr 163 (1): 38–44

Bredella MA, Tirman PF, Peterfy CG et al. (1999) Accuracy of T2-weighted fast spin-echo MR imaging with fat saturation in detecting cartilage defects in the knee: comparison with arthroscopy in 130 patients. AJR Am J Roentgenol 172 (4): 1073–1080

De Smet AA, Ilahi OA, Graf BK (1997) Untreated osteochondritis dissecans of the femoral condyles: prediction of patient outcome using radiographic and MR findings. Skeletal Radiol 26 (8): 463–467

Lang P, Grampp S, Vahlensieck M et al. (1995) Spontane Osteonekrose des Kniegelenkes: MRT im Vergleich zur CT, Szintigraphie und Histologie. Rofo Fortschr Geb Röntgenstr Neuen Bildgeb Verfahr 162 (6): 469–477

Lotke PA, Ecker ML, Barth P, Lonner JH (2000) Subchondral magnetic resonance imaging changes in early osteoarthrosis associated with tibial osteonecrosis. Arthroscopy 16 (1): 76–81

Marti CB, Rodriguez M, Zanetti M, Romero J (2000) Spontaneous osteonecrosis of the medial compartment of the knee: a MRI follow-up after conservative and operative treatment, preliminary results. Knee Surg Sports Traumatol Arthrosc 8 (2): 83–88

Mori R, Ochi M, Sakai Y, Adachi N, Uchio Y (1999) Clinical significance of magnetic resonance imaging (MRI) for focal chondral lesions. Magn Reson Imaging 17 (8): 1135–1140

Parker RK, Ross GJ, Urso JA (1997) Transient osteoporosis of the knee. Skeletal Radiol 26 (5): 306–309

Pham XV, Monteiro I, Judet O, Sissakian JF, Plantin P, Aegerter P, Le Parc JM (1999) Magnetic resonance imaging changes in periarticular soft tissues during flares of medial compartment knee osteoarthritis. Preliminary study in 10 patients. Rev Rhum Engl Ed 66 (7–9): 398–403

Pomeranz SJ (1991) Orthopaedic MRI. JB Lippincott, Philadelphia, pp 87, 98–101, 115

Rubin DA, Harner CD, Costello JM (2000) Treatable chondral injuries in the knee: frequency of associated focal subchondral edema. AJR Am J Roentgenol 174 (4): 1099–1106

Schneider T, Fink B, Jerosch J, Assheuer J, Ruther W (1998) The value of magnetic resonance imaging as postoperative control after arthroscopic treatment of osteochondritis dissecans. Arch Orthop Trauma Surg 117 (4–5): 235–239

Smith DS, Sharp DC, Resendes M (1994) MRI of healing osteochondritis dissecans fragment with absorbable pins. J Comput Assist Tomogr 18 (5): 832–833

Waldschmidt JG, Braunstein EM, Buckwalter KA (1999) Magnetic resonance imaging of osteoarthritis. Rheum Dis Clin North Am 25 (2): 451–465

Waterton JC, Solloway S, Foster JE et al. (2000) Diurnal variation in the femoral articular cartilage of the knee in young adult humans. Magn Reson Med 43 (1): 126–132

Fig. 14.1 a, b. Osteochondritis dissecans, grade I, posterior lateral condyle (17-year-old female)

a Sagittal T1; **b** sagittal T2*: Discreet signal decrease of subchondral bone in posterior margin of lateral condyle on T1-weighting with a slight signal increase on relative T2-weighting (*arrows*). No chondral defect

a

b

Fig. 14.2 a, b. Osteochondritis dissecans, grade I, medial condyle (7-year-old girl)

a Sagittal T1; **b** sagittal T2*: Band-to bowl-shaped subchondral area of decreased intensity of posterior parts of the pressure-bearing zone of the medial condyle on T1-weighting with a slightly increased signal on relative T2-weighting (*arrows*). Intact articular cartilage

a

b

Fig. 14.3 a, b. Largely consolidated osteochondritis dissecans, grade II, medial condyle (12-year-old boy)

a Sagittal T1; b sagittal T2*: Only T1-weighted image depicts subchondral lesion in the area of the pressure-bearing zone of the medial condyle delineated by a curved black line (*arrow*). For the most part, lesion shows only mild hypointensity. No signal increase on relative T2-weighting. Intact articular cartilage

a

b

Fig. 14.4a, b. Osteochondritis dissecans, grade II – III, posterior medial condyle (14-year-old boy)

a Sagittal T1; **b** sagittal T2*: Ovoid bone fragment with normal bone signal nearly completely delineated by delicate black margin in the posterior part of the pressure-bearing zone of the medial condyle. Mild signal increase of the surrounding cleft on relative T2-weighting (*arrow*). Intact articular cartilage

a

b

c

d

Fig. 14.5 a–d. Osteochondritis dissecans, grade II–III, medial condyle (24-year-old male)

a Coronal T1; **c** sagittal T1; **b** axial T2*; **d** sagittal T2*: Almost completely delineated ovoid bone fragment of low signal intensity in both sequences located laterally in the base area of the medial condyle. Connected to native bone only by a tiny bony lamella anteriorly (*arrowhead* in **d**). No displacement. Thinning of articular cartilage. Hypointensity on T1-weighting consistent with regressive changes. Sclerosis of mouse bed and bone fragment clearly delineated by black margin and fluid, respectively

Fig. 14.6. Femorotibial chondro-malacia, grade I, medial compart-ment; tear of medial meniscal posterior horn partly outside image (31-year-old male)

Sagittal T2*: Thickening of articular cartilage overlying pressure-bearing zone of medial condyle and of medial tibial plateau (*arrows*). Discreet contour incongruence of superior surface of medial meniscal posterior horn (*arrowhead*). Slight joint effusion

Fig. 14.7. Femorotibial chondro-malacia, grade I – II, medial compartment; tear of medial meniscal posterior horn, grade III (52-year-old male)

Sagittal T2*: Thickening of articular cartilage overlying pressure-bearing zone of medial condyle with slightly decreased signal intensity of surface. Slight irregularity of opposed tibial articular cartilage (*arrows*). Medial meniscal posterior horn abnormally flattened with superior surface defect in far posterior portion (*arrowhead*). Slight to moderate reactive effusion

a

b

Fig. 14.8 a, b. Femorotibial chondromalacia, grade III; joint effusion with loose bodies/joint chondromas (39-year-old male)

a Sagittal T2*; **b** axial T2*: Highly irregular articular cartilage in medial compartment. Extensive exposure of underlying bone in the area of the pressure-bearing zone of the medial condyle (*arrow*). Faintly discernible bony excrescence at anterior margin of medial condyle. Central meniscal signal increases without tear. Moderate joint effusion with disc-shaped loose bodies of low to absent signal intensity in the medial supra-patellar recess (*arrowheads*)

Fig. 14.9 a, b. Femorotibial chondromalacia, grade IV, in a patient with severe, activated gonarthritis (74-year-old male)

a Sagittal T1; b sagittal T2*: Extensive, almost bandlike, delicately septated subchondral signal intensity decreases of opposed femorotibial areas on T1-weighting (**a**) with pronounced signal increase on relatively T2-weighted image (**b**) (*arrows*). Completely consumed articular cartilage. Very pronounced narrowing of joint cleft. No meniscal structures identified. Markedly narrowed femoropatellar joint cleft at the margin of the respective image (*arrowheads*), articular cartilage likewise completely consumed but without subchondral reaction. Partly hypertrophic bony excrescences, most pronounced on anterior condyles. Obliquely sectioned osteophytes mimicking isolated anterior fragments. Slight joint effusion

Fig. 14.10. Femorotibial chondromalacia, grade IV, medial compartment, in a patient with activated arthritis; degenerative meniscal tears with almost completely consumed medial meniscus (81-year-old female)

Coronal T1: Subchondral signal reductions of opposed areas of the medial compartment with medial joint cleft narrowing, less pronounced peripherally. No normal meniscal signal. Centrally increased signal of lateral meniscus, consistent with central degeneration without tear. Slightly distended medial collateral ligament. Obesity

Fig. 14.11 a, b. Spontaneous osteonecrosis of medial condyle in a patient with slight arthritis and degenerative tears of medial meniscal posterior horn; capsular edema, joint effusion, Baker's cyst (79-year-old female)

a Sagittal T1; **b** sagittal T2*: Extensive wavelike signal decrease with a surrounding black margin of the pressure-bearing zone of the medial condyle on T1-weighted image (**a**). Relatively T2-weighted image shows markedly hyperintense lesion (**b**). Elevated cortical lamella centrally. Abnormal central signal increase of medial meniscal posterior horn on both sequences – contour disruption not depicted on images. Relatively T2-weighted image shows pronounced joint effusion of high signal intensity including Baker's cyst at the slightly hyperintense posterior capsular margin

Fig. 14.12 a, b. Spontaneous osteonecrosis of medial condyle/ chondromalacia, grade II (to IV); tear of medial meniscal posterior horn, grade III – IV; reactive effusion (58-year-old male)

a Sagittal T1; **b** sagittal T2*: T1-weighted image showing curved signal decrease of the pressure-bearing zone of the medial condyle, partly demarcated by hypointense to absent signal intensity. Markedly increased signal intensity of the lesion with some roundish areas of more pronounced hyperintensity posteriorly (*arrowhead*) on relative T2-weighting. Abnormal signal increase of medial meniscal posterior horn on both sequences with multiple contour disruptions, most conspicuous on relative T2-weighting (**b**). Irregular, moderately thinned articular cartilage on medial condyle. Pronounced joint effusion and small Baker's cyst showing increased signal intensity on relatively T2-weighted image

a

b

c

d

Fig. 14.13 a – d. Spontaneous osteonecrosis of medial condyle; tear of medial meniscal posterior horn (80-year-old female)

a, b Sagittal T1; **c, d** sagittal T2*: T1-weighted images show extensive, slightly undulated area of decreased signal in basal parts of medial condyle, partly delineated by absent signal intensity (**b**). Pronounced signal increase of this area with a large anterior extension stretching proximally (*arrows*) on relative T2-weighting. Flattening of the cortex and delicate contour disruptions in the area of the pressure-bearing zone. Articular cartilage markedly thinned. Slight osteochondral separation (**d**). Nonvisualization of medial meniscal posterior horn. Slight joint effusion

a

b

c

d

Fig. 14.14a–d. Osteonecrotic area of posterior medial condyle; degenerative tear of medial meniscal posterior horn (60-year-old female)

a Coronal T1; c sagittal T1; b axial T2*; d sagittal T2*: T1-weighted images (a, c) showing subchondral area of decreased signal intensity in posterior medial condyle (*arrow*). The lesion is partly septated by delicate black lamellae and delineated by margin of absent signal intensity. Much less pronounced corresponding changes also in anterior aspect of medial condyle (*arrowhead*). Pronounced signal increases of these areas on relative T2-weighting (b, d). Thinning of articular cartilage in medial compartment with extensive exposure of underlying bone in the area of the pressure-bearing zone. Medial meniscal posterior horn abnormally increased in signal, in part barely discernible, and showing pronounced contour disruptions (a, c, d)

a

b

c

Fig. 14.15 a – c. Bone contusion of lateral condyle; reactive effusion-distortion 6 weeks earlier (47-year-old female)

a Coronal T1; b sagittal T1; c sagittal T2*: Extensive mild signal decrease of posterior medial condyle on T1-weighted images (a, b) and increased signal intensity on relative T2-weighting – indicated by *arrow* in each image. No cortical disruption, no chondral defect. Intact lateral meniscus with only slight central signal increase/degeneration of anterior horn. Slight reactive effusion. Osteonecrosis is unlikely in the absence of spongy bone reduction

15 Bone Infarct

15.1 Technique and Method

In general, MRI of bone infarcts typically occurring in the diaphyseal and metaphyseal bone of the distal femur requires acquisition of additional sequences proximal to the knee joint.

The lesions can be identified and delineated using fat-suppressed sequences and T1-weighted sequences. Administration of an intravenous contrast medium may in some cases be necessary to differentiate bone infarcts from enchondromas or bone cysts.

15.2 Normal MRI Appearance

The normal marrow space in the area of the distal femoral diaphysis and metaphysis is of homogeneous hyperintensity and clearly delineated from the surrounding black compact bone on T1-weighted imaging.

15.3 Pathomechanism

Avascular bone necrosis.

15.4 Pathophysiology

Bone infarcts are distinguished from other avascular osteonecroses which predominantly occur subchondrally at the convex ends of bones in that they affect the metaphyseal area and marrow.

The knee is a preferred site of occurrence (metaphyseal bone of the proximal tibia and distal femur). Bone infarcts are frequently multiple in location and are occasionally observed in association with barotrauma, long-term cortisone therapy, and certain metabolic disorders.

15.5 MRI Signs of Abnormal Findings

Early Bone Infarct

Early bone infarct is depicted as a longitudinally oriented, frequently lobulated, intramedullary area of decreased signal intensity on T1-weighted images and increased signal on T2-weighted images, partly delineated by a black margin. This appearance may occasionally make it difficult to differentiate a bone infarct from enchondroma. Such inconclusive cases require radiographic control or possibly follow-up by MRI (Figs. 15.1 and 15.2).

Old Bone Infarct

In more long-standing bone infarct, sclerosis or ossification has already progressed to the center of the necrotic area as indicated by signal intensity isointense with marrow on T1-weighted images. Marginal sclerosis or calcifications persist as serpiginous areas with no signal.

Relatively T2-weighted imaging shows almost no signal intensity increase of the central area at this stage. This appearance represents conclusive evidence and requires no further follow-up (Figs. 15.3 and 15.4).

15.6 Clinical Role of MRI Findings

Bone infarcts as a rule require no treatment. Their differentiation from other conditions, specifically calcifying chondromas, is important but difficult. In general, bone infarcts tend to calcify from the margin to the center and chondromas from the center to the margin.

Bony changes around the calcification (contour distention, scalloping phenomenon) are typical of enchondroma and rule out bone infarction.

MRI frequently demonstrates cartilage matrix in the immediate vicinity of calcified foci of enchondroma. In individual cases, the differential diagnosis can only be made on the basis of conventional radiographs, MR images, and possibly CT scans.

Further Reading

Bohndorf K (1991) MR-Tomographie des Skeletts und der peripheren Weichteile. Springer, Berlin Heidelberg New York Tokyo, pp 99–101

Munk PL, Helms CA, Holt RG (1989) Immature bone infarcts: findings on plain radiographs and MR-scans. AJR Am J Roentgenol 152: 547–549

Stoller DW (1997) Magnetic Resonance Imaging in Orthopaedics + Sport Medicine, 2nd edn. Lippincott-Raven, Philadelphia, p 1270

Table 15.1. Characteristic signal intensities

	T1w	T2w	T2*w	rho-w	FAT-SAT
Compact/ spongy bone	0	0	0	0	0
Marrow (yellow)	↑↑↑	↑ – ↑↑	0 – ↑	↑↑	0
Marrow (red)	↑↑	↑	↑	↑	↑ – ↑↑
Bone infarct (early)	0 – ↑	↑↑↑	↑↑ – ↑↑↑	↑↑↑	↑↑ – ↑↑↑
Bone infarct (old)	0 – ↑	↑ – ↑↑	↑	↑	↑ – ↑↑

0 No signal; ↑ low SI; ↑↑ intermediate SI; ↑↑↑ high SI.

a

b

c

d

Fig. 15.1 a–d. Bone infarct of the distal femoral metaphysis, partly active/residual edema phase (64-year-old male)

a Coronal T1; **b, c** sagittal T1; **d** sagittal T2*: Both sequences show an ovoid lesion in the distal femoral metaphysis of marrow intensity with hypointense stippling and surrounded by a low-signal serpiginous margin. On relatively T2-weighted image some isolated hyperintense areas are discernible within the lesion, predominantly posteriorly and basally (*arrows*)

a

b

c

d

Fig. 15.2 a–d. Bone infarct of central tibial metaphysis (partial edema – no other diagnostic procedures) (22-year-old male)

a Coronal T1; c sagittal T1; b axial T2*; d sagittal T2*: Ovoid lesion in the proximal tibial metaphysis with partly extensive central areas of normal marrow signal and serpiginous marginal sclerosis of absent signal intensity. Stipples and septum-like structures of reduced signal intensity also within the lesion. Only very mild additional intralesional signal decreases on T1-weighted images, especially anteriorly and laterally (arrows in a and c). Extensive hyperintensities except for central areas on relatively T2-weighted images (b, d)

Fig. 15.3 a, b. Multiple older bone infarcts of distal femur and proximal tibia – with only minimal edema near joint (17-year-old female)

a Sagittal T1; **b** sagittal T2*: Both sequences show very extensive lesions surrounded by black serpiginous margins in the distal femoral diaphysis, metaphysis, and epiphysis and in the proximal tibial metaphysis. Central signal intensity of each lesion fairly isointense to bone marrow. Only some isolated small areas near the joint show pronounced hyperintensity on relatively T2-weighted image (*arrows* in **b**)

Fig. 15.4. Bone infarct of distal femoral diaphysis/metaphysis (66-year-old male)

Sagittal; *left* T1, *right* T2*: Longitudinal, ovoid, punctiform areas with no signal in the center of the marrow space of the distal femur on both sequences. Relatively T2-weighted image shows a slight signal increase only at the medial margin of the middle third of the lesion (*arrow*)

16 Inflammatory Changes

16.1 Technique and Method

Inflammatory processes of the joint can best be evaluated using fat-suppressed and T2-weighted sequences. The most important questions to be answered by MRI pertain to the *localization* and *extension* of exudative and proliferative synovial changes.

Intravenous contrast medium administration is most useful for identifying and differentiating proliferative and destructive components.

16.2 Normal MRI Appearance

Fluid collections are also present in the normal joint, especially in infrapatellar and posterior location, while synovial proliferation is always an abnormal finding.

16.3 Pathomechanism

Soft Tissue

Soft tissue inflammation of the knee is a primary disease of the synovial membrane. Etiologically, a distinction is made between bacterial inflammation (caused by unspecific agents, tubercle bacilli, *Borrelia*, and other organisms) and nonbacterial inflammation (such as reactive arthritis, gouty arthritis, chronic polyarthritis).

Bone

The bone may likewise be affected by bacterial or nonbacterial inflammation, with bacterial processes – osteomyelitis in the strict sense of the term – being by far more common.

16.4 Pathophysiology

Soft Tissue

Soft tissue inflammation of the knee may occur as localized gonarthritis or as genicular involvement of systemic disorders. The release into the synovium of substances that are destructive to cartilage and the proliferation of the synovial membrane in the course of inflammation lead to secondary destruction of cartilage and subchondral bone.

Bone

Based on the pathway of spread of the infection, a distinction is made between hematogenous and exogenous osteomyelitis. The localization of exogenous osteomyelitis is determined by the type of the direct pathway of infection.

Hematogenous osteomyelitis predominantly affects metaphyseal (diaphyseal) bone areas. Whether there will also be joint space involvement primarily depends on the patient's age (Figs. 16.8 and 16.9).

Osteomyelitis in neonates rapidly spreads to the joint space along the epimetaphyseal vessels still present at this age.

In juvenile hematogenous osteomyelitis, the growth plate presents an insurmountable barrier to pathogen spread. Invasion of the joint space is delayed and occurs through invasion via the cortex with subsequent subperiosteal infection of intracapsular bone areas (distal femoral metaphysis).

In adults there may again be rapid spread of the infection along the epimetaphyseal vascular connection reestablished by closure of the physis.

16.5 MRI Signs of Abnormal Findings

Soft Tissue (Joint Space)

Exudative synovitis is associated with increased volumes of joint fluid depicted on T2-weighted images as areas of increased signal intensity. Such excess fluid is predominantly seen in the supra- and parapatellar region in early disease and later also extends to central and posterior areas of the joint. At this later stage, there is also frequent fluid diffusion into the area of Hoffa's fat pad as well as into periarticular muscle and subcutaneous soft tissue (Figs. 16.1 and 16.2).

In *proliferative synovitis* a distinction is made between thickening of the synovial membrane confined to the joint space and an aggressive destructive form possibly extending subchondrally. Both forms of synovial proliferation show pronounced contrast enhancement (Figs. 16.3–16.7).

Subchondral bone defects associated with destructive synovitis are markedly hypointense on unenhanced T1-weighted images and have an increased signal intensity on relatively and purely T2-weighted images. The pronounced enhancement after contrast medium administration may in part obscure the bony defects.

Since proliferated synovial membranes likewise contain excess amounts of water, it may be difficult to distinguish proliferative and exudative components on the basis of T2-weighted images alone because both the thickened membrane and effusion are markedly hyperintense.

Optimal differentiation of the two components, on the other hand, is achieved by intravenous contrast medium administration, which will produce pronounced enhancement of the proliferative membrane on T1-weighted images.

Subchondral erosion and destruction tend to occur earlier in bacterial infection than in chronic inflammatory conditions such as rheumatic diseases. Joint tuberculosis as a very rare specific form of infection does not have a specific MRI appearance, presenting with exudative and proliferative components and slowly progressive destruction.

Bone

Like malignant tumors, inflammatory (osteomyelitic) foci confined to the bone are depicted as markedly hypointense lesions in the marrow on T1-weighted images and show pronounced hyperintensity on relatively T2-weighted and fat-suppressed images (Fig. 16.8).

In more extensive disease, larger foci containing isolated necrotic bone sequestra of lower signal intensity accompanied by thinning of the cortex or contour disruption may be seen. With fistulation, there will be inflammatory involvement of periosseous soft tissue, often seen as cuff-like areas with signal changes similar to those in intraosseous lesions (Figs. 16.9 and 17.21).

On contrast-enhanced imaging, all inflammatory lesions except for liquefied areas and the content of abscesses show pronounced enhancement, resulting in improved assessment of extraosseous manifestations while intraosseous lesions tend to be obscured.

16.6 Clinical Role of MRI Findings

Soft Tissue

MRI does not provide a specific diagnosis of inflammatory conditions of the knee but is well suited to differentiate free fluid from synovial proliferation and allows for the early identification of secondary chondral/subchondral destruction.

Bone

A specific diagnosis of bacterial and nonbacterial inflammatory bone changes can only be made in conjunction with the clinical findings. When an infection is diagnosed clinically, MRI is useful in assessing the extent of the process but is limited in that it cannot distinguish, for instance, a bacterial inflammatory lesion proper from perifocal edema. However, MRI does have an important role in noninvasively assessing involvement of the joint space.

Table 16.1. Characteristic signal intensities

	T1w	T2w	T2*w	rho-w	FAT-SAT
Effusion (serous)	0 – ↑	↑↑↑	↑↑↑	↑ – ↑↑	↑↑↑
Synovial proliferation					
precontrast	0 – ↑	↑ – ↑↑	↑↑	↑↑	↑ – ↑↑
postcontrast	↑↑ – ↑↑↑	↑↑	↑↑	↑↑	↑ – ↑↑

0 No signal; ↑ low SI; ↑↑ intermediate SI; ↑↑↑ high SI.

Further Reading

Forslind K, Larsson EM, Johansson A, Svensson B (1997) Detection of joint pathology by magnetic resonance imaging in patients with early rheumatoid arthritis. Br J Rheumatol 36 (6): 683–688

Gaffney K, Cookson J, Blades S, Coumbe A, Blake D (1998) Quantitative assessment of the rheumatoid synovial microvascular bed by gadolinium-DTPA enhanced magnetic resonance imaging. Ann Rheum Dis 57 (3): 152–157

Graif M, Schweitzer ME, Marks B, Matteucci T, Mandel S (1998) Synovial effusion in reflex sympathetic dystrophy: an additional sign for diagnosis and staging. Skeletal Radiol 27 (5): 262–265

Leitch R, Walker SE, Hillard AE (1996) The rheumatoid knee before and after arthrocentesis and prednisolone injection: evaluation by Gd-enhanced MRI. Clin Rheumatol 15 (4): 358–366

McGonagle D, Gibbon W, O'Connor P, Green M, Pease C, Emery P (1998) Characteristic magnetic resonance imaging entheseal changes of knee synovitis in spondylarthropathy. Arthritis Rheum 41 (4): 694–700

McNicholas MJ, Brooksbank AJ, Walker CM (1999) Observer agreement analysis of MRI grading of knee osteoarthritis. J R Coll Surg Edinb 44 (1): 31–33

Oliver C, Watt I (1996) Intravenous MRI contrast enhancement of inflammatory synovium: a dose study. Br J Rheumatol 35 (3): 31–35

Ostergaard M, Stoltenberg M, Henriksen O, Lorenzen I (1996) Quantitative assessment of synovial inflammation by dynamic gadolinium-enhanced magnetic resonance imaging. A study of the effect of intra-articular methylprednisolone on the rate of early synovial enhancement. Br J Rheumatol 35 (1): 50–59

Ostergaard M, Stoltenberg M, Lovgreen Nielsen P, Volck B, Jensen CH, Lorenzen I (1997) Magnetic resonance imaging-determined synovial membrane and joint effusion volumes in rheumatoid arthritis and osteoarthritis: comparison with the macroscopic and microscopic appearance of the synovium. Arthritis Rheum 40 (10): 1856–1867

Ostergaard M, Stoltenberg M, Lovgreen Nielsen P, Volck B, Sonne Holm, Lorenzen I (1998) Quantification of synovitis by MRI: correlation between dynamic and static gadolinium-enhanced magnetic resonance imaging and microscopic and macroscopic signs of synovial inflammation. Magn Reson Imaging 16 (7): 743–754

Poleksic L, Musikic P, Zdravkovic D, Watt I, Bacic G (1996) MRI evaluation of the knee in rheumatoid arthritis. Br J Rheumatol 35 (3): 36–39

Ramsey SE, Cairns RA, Cabral DA, Malleson PN, Bray HJ, Petty RE (1999) Knee magnetic resonance imaging in childhood chronic monarthritis. J Rheumatol 367: 158–164

Rand T, Imhof H, Czerny C, Breitenseher M, Machold K, Turetschek K, Trattnig S (1999) Discrimination between fluid, synovium, and cartilage in patients with rheumatoid arthritis: contrast enhanced spin echo versus non-contrast-enhanced fat-suppressed gradient echo MR imaging. Clin Radiol 54 (2): 107–110

Takeuchi K, Inoue H, Yoliyama Y, Senda M, Ota Y, Abe N, Nishida K (1998) Evaluation of rheumatoid arthritis using a scoring system devised from magnetic resonance imaging of rheumatoid knees. Acta Med Okayama 52 (4): 211–224

Zanetti M, Bruder E, Romero J, Hodler J (2000) Bone marrow edema pattern in osteoarthritic knees: correlation between MR imaging and histologic findings. Radiology 215 (3): 835–840

a

b

Fig. 16.1 a, b. Exudative synovitis in infancy (2 $1/2$-year-old boy)

a Sagittal T1; **b** sagittal T2*: Pronounced joint effusion with high signal intensity on relatively T2-weighted image (**b**). Very thick articular cartilage normal for age but showing minimal contour irregularity in the area of the anterior femur. Just barely discernible signal increase of the distal femoral metaphysis on relative T2-weighting as a weak concomitant reaction. Small extension of Baker's cyst with fluid signal in popliteal area

Fig. 16.2 a–d. Predominantly exudative arthritis with slight proliferative component, no chondral erosion (44-year-old male)

a Sagittal T1; **b** sagittal T2*; **c, d** contrast-enhanced sagittal T1: Relatively T2-weighted image (**b**) showing extensive hyperintensity indicating marked increase in joint fluid volume with conspicuous, septum-like structures in the suprapatellar recess (*arrow*). Unenhanced T1-weighted image (**a**) without any suggestive abnormalities. Following contrast medium administration, however, pronounced synovial enhancement including the septum-like suprapatellar structures (*arrows* in **c** and **d**)

a

b

c

d

Fig. 16.3 a–d. Considerable synovitis with pannus in retropatellar area and posterior joint recess, psoriasis (27-year-old female)

a Sagittal T1; **b** contrast-enhanced sagittal T1: Unenhanced T1-weighted image only shows pronounced suprapatellar effusion of decreased signal intensity and slight thickening of synovial structures, most conspicuous directly anterior to the femur (*arrow* in **a**). Contrast-enhanced image shows pronounced synovial enhancement including the prefemoral focal thickenings (*black arrow* in **b**) but above all also pronounced enhancement of the retropatellar area and of the entire posterior joint recess (*white arrow* in **b**)

c Sagittal T2*; **d** axial T2*: Considerable joint effusion with increased signal intensity on T2-weighted images. Preformal focal thickenings depicted as hypointense gaps. Pannus in the retropatellar area and posterior joint recess is poorly delineated due to just slightly lower signal intensity than suprapatellar joint fluid

Fig. 16.4 a – f. Destructive gonarthritis with pannus formation (exudative/proliferative synovitis with meniscal, cruciate ligament, and bony defects; 18-year-old female)

a Coronal T1: Small bowl-shaped contour defect of both the femur in the laterobasal aspect of the lateral condyle and of the medial tibial plateau adjacent to the base of the medial eminence tubercle (*arrowheads*). Very extensive filling of the joint space nearly isointense with soft tissue including the intercondylar fossa and the lateral joint recess. Cruciate ligament structures poorly delineated.

b Sagittal T2*: Markedly hyperintense joint effusion. Defects of posterior aspect of Hoffa's fat pad. Abnormally thickened silhouette of the anterior cruciate ligament with fibers in posterior portion no longer clearly discernible (*arrow*)

Fig. 16.4 c – f see p. 244

c

d

e

f

Fig. 16.4c–f. Destructive gonarthritis with pannus formation (exudative/proliferative synovitis with meniscal, cruciate ligament, and bony defects; 18-year-old female)

c, d Unenhanced sagittal T1; **e, f** contrast-enhanced sagittal T1: Wedge- to bowl-shaped surface defect of the medial tibial plateau near eminence (**c, d**). Fluid to soft tissue signal intensity throughout the joint space, in particular also in the vicinity of the poorly delineated anterior cruciate ligament (*arrow* in **c**). After contrast medium administration, there is massive enhancement of the entire posterior joint recess in the vicinity of the posterior cruciate ligament obscuring most of the anterior cruciate. Additional enhancement also at the posterior margin of Hoffa's fat pad with the exception of isolated fluid-containing parts (*arrows* in **e, f**). Delicate synovial enhancement of prefemoral area and suprapatellar recess

Fig. 16.5 a, b. Destructive arthritis with formation of new cartilage (12-year-old girl)

a Coronal T1; **b** sagittal T1: Curved cortical defects of the medial condyle epiphysis basomedially with less pronounced defects also in the anterior aspect of the medial tibial plateau (*arrows*). Defect-induced widening of the antero-medial joint space. Some residual cartilage of lower signal intensity in the inflamed area

a

b

Fig. 16.6. Arthritis of proximal tibiofibular joint (63-year-old female)

Sagittal; *left* T1, *right* T2*: Extensive contour irregularities of the proximal tibiofibular joint with opposing bone areas showing mild, partly bandlike, signal reduction on T1-weighted image and increased signal on relative T2-weighting (*arrows*). Markedly increased joint fluid volume of high signal intensity on relative T2-weighting (*right image*)

a

b

Fig. 16.7 a, b. Older bone infarcts/inflammatory subcortical lesion of anterior distal femur and patella; status post recurrent arthritis (58-year-old male)

a Sagittal T1; **b** sagittal T2*: T1-weighted image showing mild, partly serpiginous, signal decreases in the distal femoral metaphysis with a more extensive subchondral area of lower intensity at the anterior margin of the lateral condyle. Hardly any signal decreases of patella and proximal tibial plateau, whereas relatively T2-weighted image shows pronounced signal increase of central areas of superior patella (*arrow*) as well as slightly increased signal of the anterior margin of the lateral condyle. The distal femoral metaphysis predominantly shows decreased signal intensity with only some areas of slightly increased signal. Hardly any joint effusion. Slight patella alta

Fig. 16.8 a, b. Chronic femoral osteomyelitis with sequestration and involvement of knee joint (55-year-old female)

a Sagittal T1; b sagittal T2*:
T1-weighted image showing pronounced longitudinally oriented hypointensity of the distal femoral metaphysis with extensions to the anterior margin of the lateral condyle. Some islands of marrow intensity within the hypointense metaphyseal lesion and isolated larger area proximally (*arrow*).
On relative T2-weighting, the metaphyseal/epiphyseal lesion shows slightly heterogeneous hyperintensity with a roundish signal reduction proximally (*arrow*). Markedly hyperintense joint effusion

a

b

a

b

c

d

Fig. 16.9 a–d. Chronic osteomyelitis of distal femur; cloaca, sequestration, and subcutaneous fistula after previous fixateur externe (32-year-old female)

a Coronal T2*: Laterally increasing wedge-shaped bone defect of heterogeneous hyperintensity in the supra- and intracondylar aspect of the distal femur with a street-like extension to the lateral subcutaneous fatty tissue. Focal signal voids representing metal artifacts in the meta- and epiphyseal bone and partial thickening of cortical structures, due to sclerosis and metal artifacts

b Sagittal T1: Wedge-shaped to tubular contour defect of the anterior margin of the lateral condyle with a connection to the retropatellar joint space, depicted as marked hypointensity with some isolated marginal areas of marrow intensity basally (*arrows*)

c Unenhanced coronal T1; **d** contrast-enhanced coronal T1: Unenhanced image depicts wedge-shaped defect zone in lateral aspect of distal femur with hypointense signal intensity and central areas of moderately hypointense to intermediate signal intensity. Small isolated bone parts, in particular laterobasally (*arrowhead*). Contrast-enhanced image shows pronounced enhancement of the defect including subcutaneous area with some roundish filling defects (*arrows*) representing debris

17 Tumors and Tumorlike Lesions

17.1 Technique and Method

Tumors and tumorlike lesions are frequently discovered incidentally in patients undergoing MRI of the knee for other reasons. Further MRI assessment therefore depends on the localization and extent of such lesions.

17.2 Normal MRI Appearance

Normal bone marrow is hyperintense on T1-weighted images (rule of thumb: "White is right"). Hematopoietic zones in the metaphyseal and diaphyseal marrow space may have a mildly hypointense signal on both T1-weighted images and on relatively or purely T2-weighted images.

Cortical bone has absent signal intensity in all sequences. Tendinous structures and the menisci are typically hypointense in both sequences. Normal muscle is of intermediate signal intensity.

17.3 Pathophysiology

Juxta-articular Bone Lesions

Tumors and tumorlike lesions of the bone have a predilection for the segments of the long bones near the knee (in order of decreasing frequency: femur, tibia, and fibula), affecting predominantly the metaphysis.

Purely epiphyseal tumors limited to the immediately periarticular bone area are rare. Among the benign tumors, only chondroblastomas are of this type. Meta- and epiphyseal extension may be seen in all malignant tumors as well as in giant cell tumors and aneurysmal bone cysts.

Soft Tissue Lesions

Soft tissue lesions around the knee are uncommon. Along with well-defined tumor entities such as neurinomas or lipomas, which occur very rarely in the soft tissue structures of the knee, the following soft tissue tumors and tumorlike conditions may be encountered in the knee:

- Hemangioma.
- Villonodular synovitis.
- Focal nodular synovitis (synovioma).
- Articular chondromatosis.

Hemangioma. This is a benign tumor with proliferation of endothelial cells. Hemangiomas predominantly affect the skin but may also be found in any other organ as well as in and around the knee.

Hemangiomas of the knee present with swelling that characteristically increases with the leg lowered and decreases when the leg is elevated. The soft tissue changes may be accompanied by periosteal reactions and periarticular osteolysis.

Intra-articular hemangiomas lead to recurrent hemorrhagic joint effusion with the risk of secondary arthritis and must therefore be removed surgically.

Careful preoperative assessment is important, in particular when the intervention is performed endoscopically, to preclude the risk of intraoperative bleeding complications.

Villonodular Synovitis. Pigmented villonodular synovitis is a chronic tumorous proliferation of the synovial membrane. Typically, villonodular synovitis is monoarticular, affecting the knee in 80% of all cases.

The etiology of villonodular synovitis continues to be controversial; it may represent a benign synovial neoplasm or a reactive process induced by some unknown agent.

The chronic tumorous proliferations of the synovial membrane induce recurrent intra-articular hemorrhage, resulting in pronounced hemosiderin deposition in the deep layers of the capsule.

Pigmented villonodular synovitis extends throughout the joint and leads to extensive secondary destruction of articular cartilage that may also involve the subchondral bone.

Focal Nodular Synovitis (Synovioma). This is a strictly circumscribed process of the synovial membrane characterized by the presence of one or several adjacent nodules in an otherwise normal membrane.

Focal nodular synovitis is regarded by some as a harmless variant of (aggressive) pigmented villonodular synovitis, by others as an independent disease entity.

Articular Chondromatosis. Chondromatosis of the joint is most likely not a genuine tumor but is assumed to be caused by metaplastic differentiation of fibroblasts into chondroblasts with subsequent tumorlike proliferation of cartilage.

As a result of this process, large numbers of chondromas arise in the synovial membrane. Chondromas that have undergone mineralization are also detectable by conventional radiographs. Etiologically, the disorder is attributed to both exogenous and endogenous factors.

Initially embedded in the synovial membrane, the chondromas develop into the joint space until only a small stalk connects them to the membrane. They may also be expelled into the joint space as loose bodies.

Prompt removal of such intra-articular loose bodies is necessary to prevent secondary damage to the articular cartilage. Since chondromatosis is a primary disorder of the synovial membrane, extensive synovectomy with removal of the triggering agent is important.

17.4 MRI Signs of Abnormal Findings

Regarding the *specific diagnosis* of bone tumors, MRI is generally not superior to conventional radiographs, especially since the latter have the added advantage of clearly identifying calcifications.

A specific tumor diagnosis is primarily based on the shape, delineation, and location of the lesion as well as on the patient's age.

In terms of differentiating benign from malignant lesions, MRI is again not necessarily superior to conventional radiography. However, with its excellent soft tissue contrast, it is clearly superior to both conventional radiography and CT in assessing *lesion extent.*

MRI criteria for benign lesions are the same as in conventional radiography. These include good delineation of the lesion and/or presence of marginal sclerosis, depicted as absent signal intensity. Moreover, the absence of signal increases on relatively T2-weighted images may likewise suggest a benign lesion. Contrast enhancement, on the other hand, is inconclusive.

MRI criteria for malignant lesions are poor delineation of the lesion, cortical erosions, and extraosseous extension with infiltration of soft tissue structures including muscle. It is in the assessment of such extraosseous infiltration that additional contrast-enhanced imaging may be useful.

Given the multitude of tumors and tumorlike lesions that can involve the knee, the characteristics of only the most important ones are briefly outlined below.

Juxta-articular Bone Lesions

Osteocartilaginous Exostosis (Osteochondroma). Characterized by circumscribed protrusion of bony structures. Benign exostosis is of uniformly high signal intensity isointense with marrow on T1-weighted images and shows no signal increase on relative T2-weighting.

Abnormal signal decreases on T1-weighted images or increases on relative T2-weighting indicate active disease and require follow-up to check for potential malignant transformation. The thickness of the typical cartilage cap (increased signal on T2-weighting) is another prognostic indicator of further growth (Figs. 17.1 – 17.3).

Nonossifying Bone Fibroma. Typically located eccentrically in the metaphysis and contiguous with cortical bone surrounded by margins of absent signal intensity. Central hyperintensity on relatively T2-weighted images in the active state.

Most bone fibromas recede spontaneously (with complete regression especially after puberty) with a gradual return to normal marrow signal of the hypointense central signal on T1-weighted images and the increased signal on relative T2-weighting (Figs. 17.4–17.6).

Chondroma. Roundish lesions of marked hypointensity on T1-weighted images and hyperintensity on relative T2-weighting. Depiction of central or marginal areas of no signal suggests calcification and requires radiographic control. Differential diagnosis: early bone infarct (Figs. 17.7–17.12).

Chondroblastoma. Typically restricted to epiphysis. Well-defined lesion with hypointense signal on T1-weighted images and moderate to marked hyperintensity on relative T2-weighting, partly surrounded by margin of no signal.

Giant Cell Tumor. Likewise epiphyseal in location, typically in the immediate vicinity of the epiphyseal line, but may show extension to metaphysis. Hypointense on T1-weighted image, hyperintense on relatively T2-weighted image, frequently with slightly inhomogeneous signal pattern.

Aneurysmal Bone Cyst. Typically metaphyseal, rarely epiphyseal or diaphyseal in location, sparing the epiphyseal line. Similar signal characteristics as enchondroma, but much more homogeneous and typically of somewhat higher intensity on T1-weighted image due to blood components. May show pronounced septation or occasionally peripheral hemosiderin deposits appearing as signal voids (Fig. 17.13).

Juvenile Bone Cyst. Same location and signal characteristics as aneurysmal cyst but with little or no septation (Fig. 17.14).

Bone Metastasis/Primary Bone Sarcoma. Markedly hypointense signal on T1-weighting and hyperintensity on relatively and purely T2-weighted images, possibly with signs of destruction (Figs. 17.15, 17.16, and 17.19).

These tumors must be differentiated from systemic diseases with diffuse bone marrow involvement (such as leukemia) and anemia with replacement of fatty marrow by hematopoietic marrow, which show decreased signal intensity on T1-weighted and relatively T2-weighted images (Figs. 17.18 and 17.20).

Osteomyelitis. Intramedullary lesions with signal characteristics on T1-weighted images similar to those of malignant tumors. In addition, practically identical signal increases on relatively T2-weighted and fat-suppressed sequences.

Like malignant tumors, associated with cortical erosion, possibly with prominent cuff-like soft tissue involvement of identical signal behavior and pronounced enhancement (Fig. 17.21).

Osteomyelitic lesions often show considerable lengthwise extension but comparatively moderate destructions. Differentiation from malignant lesions frequently only possible surgically!

Soft Tissue Lesions

Intra-articular Location:

- *Synovioma*: Mass of soft tissue density with muscle signal on T1-weighted image, moderate signal increase on T2-weighting, and frequently showing contrast enhancement (see Figs. 10.7, 10.8, and 10.14).
- *Hemangioma*: Typical vessel-like tubular structures with pronounced signal increase on T2-weighting, isolated hypointense phleboliths, and marked contrast enhancement except for thrombotic areas (Figs. 17.30 and 17.31).
- *Pigmented Villonodular Synovitis*: Pseudotumorous, aggressive inflammatory condition with presence of multiple nodular structures in the joint space. Frequently very low or absent signal intensity due to hemosiderin deposition on T1- and T2-weighted images. Possibly cortical destruction. Pronounced (hemorrhagic) joint effusion. Mostly pronounced, inhomogeneous contrast enhancement after intravenous contrast medium administration (see Figs. 10.8 and 10.9; Figs. 17.32 and 17.33).

Extra-articular Location:

- Lipoma.
- Liposarcoma.
- Malignant fibrous histiocytoma.
- Fibrosarcoma.
- Synovial sarcoma.
- Rhabdomyosarcoma.
- Epithelioid sarcoma.
- Hemangiopericytoma.
- Desmoid tumor.
- Giant cell tumor of tendon sheaths.

With the exception of lipomatous lesions with fat signal (pronounced hyperintensity on T1-weighted image), soft tissue tumors are typically isointense to muscle with decreased signal intensity on T1-weighting and relative signal increases on T2-weighting and show pronounced contrast enhancement (Fig. 17.29). Conspicuously heterogeneous appearance of malignant fibrous histiocytoma. Specific lesion diagnosis generally limited, based on lesion delineation and location; only histology can provide definitive diagnosis.

These entities must be differentiated from traumatic injury (muscle strain, tear, and hemorrhage; Figs. 17.23 and 17.24), focal myositis, abscess, and granulomatous inflammation (Figs. 17.25–17.27), all of which have similar signal characteristics and may show mass effects and/or contrast medium enhancement.

17.5 Clinical Role of MRI Findings

A specific diagnosis of a bone tumor can rarely be made on the basis of the MRI findings alone. Since MRI visualizes the bone only indirectly, it is of limited value in the primary diagnostic assessment of bone tumors because harmless bone lesions such as nonossifying fibroma or osteoid osteoma may show features on MRI making them more difficult to differentiate from malignancy than by using conventional radiography or CT.

However, MRI is an excellent modality for assessing soft tissue structures and for determining tumor extension (e.g., of malignant tumors in the marrow space).

Table 17.1. Characteristic signal intensities

	T1w	T2w	T2*w	rho-w	FAT-SAT
Compact/ spongy bone	$0 - \uparrow$	0	0	0	0
Marrow (yellow)	$\uparrow\uparrow\uparrow$	$\uparrow - \uparrow\uparrow$	$0 - \uparrow$	$\uparrow\uparrow$	0
Marrow (red)	$\uparrow\uparrow$	$\uparrow$	$\uparrow$	$\uparrow$	$\uparrow - \uparrow\uparrow$
Benign bone tumors	$\uparrow - 0$	$\uparrow - \uparrow\uparrow$	$\uparrow\uparrow$	$\uparrow$	$\uparrow - \uparrow\uparrow$
Malignant bone tumors	$\uparrow - 0$	$\uparrow - \uparrow\uparrow$	$\uparrow\uparrow$	$\uparrow$	$\uparrow - \uparrow\uparrow$
Lipoma	$\uparrow\uparrow - \uparrow\uparrow\uparrow$	$\uparrow - \uparrow\uparrow$	$\uparrow$	$\uparrow\uparrow$	0

0 No signal; $\uparrow$ low SI; $\uparrow\uparrow$ intermediate SI; $\uparrow\uparrow\uparrow$ high SI.

Further Reading

Blacksin MF, Siegel JR, Benevenia J, Aisner SC (1997) Synovial sarcoma: frequency of non-aggressive MR characteristics. J Comput Assist Tomogr 21 (5): 785–789

Butler MG, Fuchigami KD, Chako A (1996) MRI of posterior knee masses. Skeletal Radiol 25 (4): 309–317

Gulati MS, Kapoor A, Maheshwari J (1999) Angiomyoma of the knee joint: value of magnetic resonance imaging. Australas Radiol 43 (3): 353–354

Hur J, Damron TA, Vermont AI, Mathur SC (1999) Fibroma of tendon sheath of the infrapatellar fat pad. Skeletal Radiol 28 (7): 407–410

Melamed JW, Martinez S, Hoffman CJ (1997) Imaging of primary multifocal osseous lymphoma. Skeletal Radiol 26 (1): 35–41

Muscolo DL, Makino A, Costa Paz M, Ayerza M (2000) Magnetic resonance imaging evaluation and arthroscopic reaction of localized pigmented villonodular synovitis of the knee. Orthopedics 23 (4): 367–369

Narvaez J, Narvaez JA, Ortega R, Juan Mas A, Roig Escofet D (1999) Lipoma arborescens of the knee. Rev Rhum Engl Ed 66 (6): 352–353

Pomeranz SJ (1991) Orthopaedic MRI. JB Lippincott, New York

Ryu KN, Jaovisidha S, Schweitzer M, Motta AO, Resnick D (1996) MR imaging of lipoma arborescens of the knee joint. AJR Am J Roentgenol 167 (5): 1229–1232

a

b

Fig. 17.1 a, b. Osteocartilaginous exostosis of proximal fibula – typical radiograph; no surgery (12-year-old boy)

a Coronal T1: Posterolateral bony protrusion of the proximal fibula with fully normal marrow signal. Small curved cartilage cap of typical intermediate signal intensity, extending almost into subcutaneous area (*arrow*)

b Axial T2*: Posterolateral protrusion of fibula with normal signal intensity and well-defined margins. Typical, smooth cartilage cap of markedly hyperintense signal (*arrow*) – fluid-containing labeling tube attached to skin

Fig. 17.2 a, b. Osteocartilaginous exostosis of posterior proximal tibia – typical radiograph; no surgery (63-year-old male)

a Sagittal T1; **b** sagittal T2*: Finger-like bony protrusion of the proximal tibial metaphysis with fully normal marrow signal (equivalent to that of native tibia on both sequences). Only tiny basal cartilage cap of weakly hyperintense signal on relatively T2-weighted image (*arrows* in **b**). Infrapatellar soft tissue edema with hyperintense signal on relatively T2-weighted image

a

b

c

Fig. 17.3a–c. Osteocartilaginous exostosis of posterior tibial plateau – typical radiograph; no surgery (33-year-old male)

a Sagittal T1: Pear-shaped bony protuberance of the posterior proximal tibial metaphysis with mostly normal marrow signal intensity equivalent to that of other tibial portions. Only some posterior subcortical areas show lower signal intensity. Impression of gastrocnemius

b Sagittal T2*; **c** axial T2*: Relatively T2-weighted images likewise show the lesion to be approximately equal in signal intensity to the bulk of the tibia. Marginal areas of lower intensity consistent with sclerosis, most prominent distally, and some barely discernible central areas of slightly higher signal intensity. Posterolateral cartilage cap thinner and slightly irregular – not suggesting malignancy but requiring follow-up. No reactive muscle involvement despite pronounced impression

Fig. 17.4a, b. Nonossifying bone fibroma of proximal tibial metaphysis – typical radiograph; no surgery (14-year-old boy)

a Sagittal T1; **b** sagittal T2*: Lesion of posterior proximal tibial metaphysis contiguous with the cortex surrounded by black margins on both sequences. Central areas of intermediate signal intensity isointense to soft tissue on T1-weighted image and moderately hyperintense on relative T2-weighting

a

b

c

d

Fig. 17.5 a – d. Nonossifying bone fibroma of distal femoral metaphysis – typical radiograph; no surgery (17-year-old male)

a Sagittal T1; **c** coronal T1: Lobulated lesion contiguous with cortex in posterolateral aspect of femur of markedly hypointense signal intensity surrounded by black margin and with some faintly seen intralesional septa

b Sagittal T2*; **d** coronal T2*: Mostly hypointense center with hyperintense anteromedial margin and black external margin

Fig. 17.6a, b. Nearly fully ossified, previously nonossifying bone fibroma of distal femoral metaphysis/diaphysis – histologically confirmed (41-year-old female)

a Coronal T1; **b** coronal T2*: T1-weighted image showing mostly normal hyperintense signal of the distal femoral metaphysis/diaphysis with only very mildly decreased signal intensity in an elongated area with curved margin (*arrows* in **a**). Relatively T2-weighted image likewise showing mostly marrow intensity except for some areas of more pronounced hypo-intensity proximally. Small hyper-intense area surrounded by black margins at the lower margin of the lesion consistent with an only dis-creet nonossified portion

a

b

Fig. 17.7 a, b. Subperiosteal chondroma of proximal tibial metaphysis – histologically confirmed (53-year-old male)

a Sagittal T1; **b** sagittal T2*: Dumbbell-shaped signal decrease in the posterior proximal tibial metaphysis contiguous with cortex. Pronounced posterior cortical thinning and minimal cortical prominence (*arrow* in **a**). Hypointense signal on T1-weighted image and markedly increased signal intensity on relatively T2-weighted image with faint marginal sclerosis (black). The patient's age and the conspicuous cortical involvement are inconsistent with nonossifying bone fibroma and the well-defined margins with a malignant lesion

Fig. 17.8 a, b. Small enchondroma of distal femoral metaphysis – discreet radiographic changes; no surgery (53-year-old male)

a Sagittal T1; **b** sagittal T2*: Small, fairly circular lesion in femoral metaphysis, surrounded by black margin on relatively T2-weighted image. Central signal of the lesion almost isointense to soft tissue on T1-weighted image and hyperintense on relative T2-weighting. Both sequences show basal areas of lower intensity indicating beginning calcification

a

b

a

b

Fig. 17.9 a, b. Enchondroma of distal femoral metaphysis – typical radiograph; no surgery (47-year-old female)

a Sagittal T1; **b** sagittal T2*: Well-defined ovoid lesion in the distal femoral metaphysis, surrounded by black margins on relatively T2-weighted image. Marked hypointensity of the lesion on T1-weighted image and slightly heterogeneous high signal intensity on relative T2-weighting with some hypointense stipples centrally. The compact appearance of the lesion and the signal pattern are not consistent with a bone infarct (cf. Fig. 15.1)

Fig. 17.10 a, b. Enchondroma of distal femoral metaphysis – typical radiograph; no surgery (51-year-old male)

a Coronal T1; **b** sagittal T2*: Ovoid lesion in the distal femoral metaphysis with slight epiphyseal extension surrounded by black margins and containing some speckled areas of no signal. Mostly hypointense centrally and nearly completely hypointense basally on T1-weighted image with marked hyperintensity of this portion on relative T2-weighting. No bone infarct (cf. Figs. 17.9 and 15.1)

a

b

a

b

Fig. 17.11 a, b. Enchondroma of proximal tibial plateau epiphysis/ metaphysis – typical radiograph, annual follow-up for 5 years; no surgery (66-year-old male)

a Sagittal T1; b sagittal T2*: Focal ovoid lesion of the tibial plateau involving the metaphysis/epiphysis, mostly surrounded by black margin. Isolated stippled areas of no signal centrally, consistent with local calcification. T1-weighted image shows grapelike solid portions and areas of soft tissue intensity mostly in anterior aspect of the lesion. Extensive, slightly heterogeneous hyperintensity on T2-weighted image. The epiphyseal extension of the lesion and the extensive portion of soft tissue intensity indicate enchondroma rather than bone infarct

Fig. 17.12 a, b. Extensive enchondroma of proximal tibial metaphysis/diaphysis – typical radiograph; no surgery (42-year-old female)

a Sagittal T1; b sagittal T2*: Elongated, ovoid mass in the center of the proximal third of the tibia. Relatively T2-weighted image shows the lesion to be surrounded by black margin and to contain punctiform areas of low to absent signal intensity, especially at the inferior margin, consistent with local calcification. Pronounced hypointensity on T1-weighted image. Despite the length of the lesion no cortical destruction, only slight curved protrusion at infero-posterior margin (*arrow* in **a**)

Fig. 17.13a, b. Aneurysmal bone cyst of distal femoral epiphysis – histologically confirmed (17-year-old female)

a Coronal T1; b axial T2*: Roundish, drop-shaped lesion in the posteromedial aspect of the distal femoral metaphysis with delicate marginal sclerosis of absent signal intensity and an intralesional signal intensity slightly above that of muscle on T1-weighted image. Markedly hyperintense signal with very discreet intralesional septation (*arrow*) on relative T2-weighting

a

b

Fig. 17.14 a, b. Bone cyst in medial aspect of medial condyle – histologically confirmed (45-year-old male)

a Coronal T1; **b** axial T2*: Ovoid lesion surrounded by black margin in the distal femoral metaphysis with epiphyseal extension. Signal intensity of the lesion on T1-weighted image only just barely above that of adjacent muscle or joint fluid with considerable hyperintensity on relative T2-weighting. Only faintly seen septation at posterior margin (*arrow*). The original MRI report discussed benign chondroblastoma and giant cell tumor with aneurysmal bone cyst components as differential diagnoses, based on the epiphyseal extension of the lesion – These tumorous lesions, however, are frequently more heterogeneous in appearance while aneurysmal bone cysts show more pronounced septation

a

b

c

Fig. 17.15 a–c. Metastasis from hypernephroma in posterior lateral condyle – histologically confirmed (46-year-old male)

a Coronal T1; **b** sagittal T1;
c sagittal T2*: Extensive mass in posterior aspect of lateral condyle, partly delineated by black margin but also showing contour irregularities and in particular pronounced reaction of surrounding bone anterosuperior to the lesion. Lesion mostly of intermediate signal intensity with slightly lower signal in the center on T1-weighting. Mild hypointensity of adjacent marrow areas. Malignancy is suggested by appearance on relatively T2-weighted image with pronounced hyperintensity of the lesion, most pronounced in the center, and by associated marrow reaction appearing as mildly increased signal intensity proximal and anterior to the lesion

Fig. 17.16 a, b. Metastasis in anterior tibial plateau, bronchial neoplasm 4 years earlier – histologically confirmed (59-year-old male)

a Coronal T1; b axial T2*: Roundish lesion in the proximal tibial plateau epiphysis with extension into the metaphysis, partly surrounded by faint marginal sclerosis of absent signal intensity but partly also showing contour irregularities. T1-weighted image shows hypointense signal of the lesion, slightly lower than that of the thigh musculature. Mild signal decrease of the area around the tibial plateau. Relatively T2-weighted image shows a markedly hyperintense lesion with irregular margin of mildly hyperintense signal intensity

Fig. 17.17. Osteosarcoma of proximal tibial metaphysis, right leg – histologically confirmed (15-year-old male)

Coronal T1: Extensive area of very low signal intensity in the right proximal tibial metaphysis with bony contour distention, pronounced cortical irregularity, and slight contour prominence medially (*arrow*). Kindly provided by K.-J. Wolf, Berlin

a

b

Fig. 17.18 a, b. Plasmocytoma of distal femoral metaphysis/ diaphysis – histologically confirmed (71-year-old female)

a Sagittal T1; **b** sagittal T2*: T1-weighted image shows elongated area of decreased signal intensity, slightly below that of surrounding muscle. Partial thinning of cortical bone without disruption (*arrowheads*). Pronounced hyperintensity with central areas of slightly lower signal intensity on relative T2-weighting (MRI preliminary diagnosis: metastasis)

Fig. 17.19 a, b. Metastasis from progressive thyroid carcinoma in distal femoral diaphysis with soft tissue infiltration – histologically confirmed (72-year-old female)

a Sagittal T1; b contrast-enhanced axial T1: Unenhanced T1-weighted image shows elongated, extensive area of decreased signal intensity in the distal femoral diaphysis with anterobasal cortical disruption (*arrowhead*). Following contrast medium administration, the tumorous lesion is much more clearly delineated from the uninvolved vastus intermedius muscle (*arrow* in **b**). Differential diagnosis: parosseous osteosarcoma

Fig. 17.20. Increased blood formation in hemolytic anemia – clinically confirmed (36-year-old female)

Sagittal T1: Massive signal decrease (equivalent to muscle) of all skeletal segments depicted including the patella. Only a small area in the distal femoral epiphysis shows high signal intensity (*arrow*)

a

b

c

d

Fig. 17.21 a–d. Tibial osteomyelitis – histologically confirmed (12-year-old boy)

a Sagittal T1: Only mildly decreased signal intensity of the marrow space of the proximal tibial metaphysis/diaphysis in the vicinity of an almost horizontal line of lower intensity (*arrow*). Cuff-like signal reduction of periosseous soft tissue (*arrowhead*)

b Axial T2*; c unenhanced axial T1; d contrast-enhanced axial T1: Slight central hyperintensity of tibial marrow space on relative T2-weighting (*arrow* in b). Lamellar periosteal elevation with extensive hyperintense reaction of surrounding soft tissue (b). Only very mild signal decrease of marrow space on precontrast T1-weighted image. Likewise conspicuous lamellar periosteal reaction and small destruction at posterior tibial margin (*arrow* in c). Postcontrast image showing pronounced enhancement of the marrow space and surrounding area including involved cortical bone. MRI differential diagnosis: Ewing's sarcoma – however, with a Ewing's sarcoma of this length there should have been more pronounced marrow signal changes as well as cortical destructions

Fig. 17.22 a, b. Paget's disease of proximal tibia – typical radiograph; histologically confirmed (56-year-old male)

a Coronal T1; **b** sagittal T1: Streaky signal decrease of the proximal tibia with extensive contour blurring laterally, proximally, and, most of all, anteriorly. Conspicuous cuff-like broadening of anterior cortical bone and soft tissue. Elevation of patellar tendon insertion (*arrow* in **b**)

a

b

Fig. 17.23 a, b. Chronic hematoma following muscle tear – histologically confirmed (52-year-old male)

a Sagittal T2; b axial T1: Extensive ovoid lesion of markedly hyperintense signal located subfascially in the anterior margin of the gastrocnemius muscle with some central areas of just slightly lower signal intensity. MRI differential diagnosis: subfascial ganglion cyst with mucous content or liposarcoma

a

b

c

d

Fig. 17.24 a – d. Partial tear of proximal gastrocnemius muscle 4 months earlier with contrast-enhancing granulation tissue – histologically confirmed (47-year-old male)

a Sagittal T2*; **b** axial T2*; **c** sagittal T1; **d** contrast-enhanced sagittal T1: Relatively T2-weighted images showing conspicuous area of increased signal intensity within proximal gastrocnemius (*arrows* in **a** and **b**). T1-weighted imaging shows normal appearance before contrast medium administration and pronounced enhancement with slightly blurred margins on postcontrast image (*arrow* in **d**). Myogenic sarcoma may show similar signal and enhancement patterns – but the lesion is typically more circular and shows much more heterogeneous signal and contrast enhancement

Fig. 17.25 a, b. Muscle irritation of proximal tibialis anterior, extensor hallucis, and extensor digitorum muscles with paresis of peroneus communis/superficialis nerve – no surgery (48-year-old male)

a, b Axial inversion recovery sequence/T2 with fat suppression: Conspicuous signal increase of anterior proximal lower leg musculature only in this sequence. No abnormalities on pre- and post-contrast T1-weighted images (*not shown*). No circumscribed mass but peroneal alteration likely due to edema (*arrows*)

Fig. 17.26 a, b. Intramuscular mass of medial proximal lower leg – histology: tumor-forming granulomatous myositis, primarily consistent with sarcoidosis (61-year-old female)

a Axial T2; **b** contrast-enhanced axial T1: Well-defined, ovoid mass in anteromedial gastrocnemius muscle (*arrows*) showing a moderately hyperintense margin on T2-weighted image (**a**) and central absence of signal on all sequences including the postcontrast study. On unenhanced T1-weighted images (*not shown*) peripheral parts of the lesion fairly similar in appearance to adjoining muscle. Pronounced enhancement of these marginal parts after contrast medium administration. No concomitant subcutaneous tissue reaction. MRI differential diagnosis: mixed fibromatous tumor; desmoid; rhabdomyosarcoma with central regression – however, the latter tumor would have much more ill-defined margins and show considerably more inhomogeneous contrast enhancement

a

b

c

Fig. 17.27 a–c. Intramusclar mass of distal thigh superolateral to condyle – histology: tumorous myositis ossificans (14-year-old girl)

a Unenhanced sagittal T1; b contrast-enhanced sagittal T1; c axial T2*: Roundish mass within femoral biceps surrounded by a shell-like margin of almost absent signal intensity suggesting marginal calcification (*arrows* in a and c). Hypointense signal, somewhat lower than that of adjoining muscle, on unenhanced T1-weighted image. Pronounced and homogeneous contrast enhancement. Markedly hyperintense signal on relative T2-weighting. MRI differential diagnosis: myxoma, leiomyoma – shell-like marginal calcification untypical with both tumors

Fig. 17.28 a, b. Subcutaneous liquefied atheroma in paratibial area – histologically confirmed (43-year-old male)

a Coronal T1; **b** axial T2*: Roundish lesion in anteromedial paratibial subcutaneous tissue with reduced signal intensity (equivalent to fluid) on T1-weighted image and marked hyperintensity on T2-weighting. Smoothly margin-ated. No reaction of surrounding structures

a

b

c

d

Fig. 17.29 a – d. Synovial sarcoma of lateral proximal lower leg, subcutaneous and intramuscular in extension – histologically confirmed; medial meniscal ganglion cyst (55-year-old female)

a Coronal T1; **b** coronal T2; **c** sagittal T2*, **d** axial T2*: Grape-shaped soft tissue mass with multiple partial septation located lateral to tibia in parafibular area. Mainly within subcutaneous tissue with extensions into peroneus longus and extensor digitorum muscles. No bone or joint involvement. Marked hypointensity, almost isointense with muscle, on T1-weighting. Intermediate signal intensity, markedly higher than that of adjacent muscle, on pure T2-weighting and pronounced hyperintensity on relative T2-weighting. Peripheral contour disruption of medial meniscal posterior horn (*arrowhead* in **a**) as an ancillary finding. Adjacent medial meniscal ganglion cyst shows marked hyperintensity compared to the less hyperintense lateral tumor manifestation on purely T2-weighted image (**b**)

Fig. 17.30 a – c. Synovial heman-gioma of suprapatellar recess – histologically confirmed (14-year-old girl)

a Coronal T1; **b** sagittal T1; **c** sagittal T2*: T1-weighted images showing grape-like lesion of decreased signal intensity within and above suprapatellar joint recess. Characteristic tubular and tortuous vascular structures, partly showing tree-like branching, depicted within the lesion. Pronounced hyperintensity on relatively T2-weighted image

a

b

c

a

b

c

Fig. 17.31 a – c. Recurrent hemangioma of left thigh, situated medially in distal half – histologically confirmed (32-year-old male)

a Contrast-enhanced coronal T1 with fat suppression: Extensive, markedly hyperintense vascular structures and convolutions in medial area of left thigh (*arrow*)

b, c Axial T2: Marked hyperintensity and partly pronounced ectasia of vessels in the vastus medialis muscle with C-shaped framing of the posteromedial femur shaft and in anterior parts of the vastus intermedius. Small black phlebolith in an ectatic vein (*arrow* in **b**). Kindly provided by M.-C. Dulce, Berlin

Fig. 17.32 a, b. Pigmented villo-nodular synovitis in retropatellar/suprapatellar area – histologically confirmed (30-year-old female)

a Sagittal T2*; **b** axial T2*: Mildly hyperintense, tortuous intra-articular lesion in retropatellar and suprapatellar recess, with synovial contact posteriorly (*arrows* in **b**). Intralesional dots of reduced signal intensity in upper and anterior margins (*arrows* in **a**). Altogether good delineation of the lesion from surrounding hyperintense fluid

a

b

c

Fig. 17.33 a – c. Pigmented villo-nodular synovitis with a 4-year history of slow progression – histologically confirmed (30-year-old male)

a Coronal T1; **b** sagittal T1: Multiple groove-like bony contour defects of femoral condyles and tibial plateau, partly surrounded by black margins. Markedly widened joint space contains multiple nodular low-intensity lesions, partly surrounded by black margins, partly showing hypointense stippling due to hemosiderin deposition. Extensive cystic fluid collections, especially in and proximal to the suprapatellar recess and in the pericapsular popliteal area

c Sagittal T2: Markedly hyperintense fluid in the suprapatellar area and popliteal soft tissue, partly interspersed with small foci of reduced signal intensity. Otherwise conspicuously low signal intensity of the joint space

Subject Index

The manufacturer's authorised representative in the EU is Springer
Nature Customer Service Centre GmbH, Europaplatz 3, 69115 Heidelberg,
Germany. If you have any concerns regarding our products, please
contact ProductSafety@springernature.com

Printed and bound by CPI Group (UK) Ltd, Croydon, CR0 4YY

28/04/2026

02098548-0002